21 Day meal planner

GI feel good
Glycemic Index

Week 1	Monday Day 1	Tuesday Day 2	Wednesday Day 3	Thursday Day 4	Friday Day 5	Saturday Day 6	Sunday Day 7
Breakfast	Swiss brown mushrooms served on wilted baby English spinach leaves	Bacon and eggs	Apricot muesli Serve of fruit	Apricot muesli	Baked beans on toast	Apricot muesli	Grilled halloumi, Roma tomatoes and prosciutto served with scrambled eggs
Lunch	Moussaka Salad with feta, cherry tomatoes and cucumber	Chicken burgers Cucumber and caper salad	Moussaka Simple rocket salad	Basmati rice salad with tomatoes, fennel and fresh herbs	Chicken burgers Salad of rocket, walnuts and feta	Tofu balls with tamarind and tomato sauce Asian salad	Basmati rice salad with tomatoes, fennel and fresh herbs Serve of fruit
	Fresh vegetable	Fresh vegetable snack					

Week 3	Monday Day 15	Tuesday Day 16	Wednesday Day 17	Thursday Day 18	Friday Day 19	Saturday Day 20	Sunday Day 21
Breakfast	Apricot muesli Serve of fruit	Swiss brown mushrooms served on wilted baby English spinach leaves	Apricot muesli Serve of fruit	Baked beans on toast	Apricot muesli Serve of fruit	Baked beans on toast	Grilled haloumi, Roma tomatoes and prosciutto served with scrambled eggs
Lunch	Spinach and ricotta tarts Cucumber and caper salad	Mushroom risotto	Spicy vegetable soup with red kidney beans and coriander	Spinach and ricotta tarts Simple rocket salad	Mushroom risotto	Egg roll ups	Salad with sardine fillets
Snack	Fresh vegetable snack Serve of cheese	Serve of fruit	Tofu balls with tamarind and tomato sauce	Fresh vegetable snack Tomato sauce with oregano Serve of cheese	Serve of fruit	Fresh vegetable snack Tomato sauce with oregano Serve of cheese	Serve of cheese
Dinner	Stir-fried seafood Salad of rocket, walnuts and feta	Barbecued fish fillets Tomato salsa	Chicken and pecan salad with lemon aioli	Beef round medallions Salsa verde salad	Fresh pasta with passata, capers and parsley	Roast lamb Roast vegetables Hollandaise sauce	Asian pork stir-fry

Protein

Carbohydrate

vegetables

Shopping and Cooking Day

	Monday Day 8	Tuesday Day 9	Wednesday Day 10	Thursday Day 11	Friday Day 12	Saturday Day 13	Sunday Day 14
Snack	snack Tomato sauce with oregano	Tomato sauce with oregano Serve of cheese	Serve of cheese Serve of nuts	Serve of fruit	Salmon muffins	Serve of fruit	Fresh vegetable snack
Dinner	Salmon muffins Tomato and basil salad	Lamb stir-fry	Spicy chicken stir-fry	Barbecued haloumi and vegetables with lemon and capers	Vegetable kebabs Tomato salsa	Fresh pasta with passata, capers and parsley tomatoes Hollandaise sauce	Roast pork Roasted Spanish onion and Roma tomatoes Hollandaise sauce

Week 2	Monday Day 8	Tuesday Day 9	Wednesday Day 10	Thursday Day 11	Friday Day 12	Saturday Day 13	Sunday Day 14
Breakfast	Apricot muesli Serve of fruit	Baked beans on toast	Swiss brown mushrooms served on wilted baby English spinach leaves	Apricot muesli Serve of fruit	Apricot muesli Serve of fruit	Baked beans on toast	Bacon and eggs
Lunch	Moussaka Salad with feta, cherry tomatoes and cucumber	Frittata with bacon and sun-dried tomatoes Tomato and basil salad	Tofu balls with tamarind and tomato sauce Asian salad	Spicy vegetable soup with red kidney beans and coriander	Frittata with bacon and sun-dried tomatoes Salad of rocket, walnuts and feta	Fresh pasta with passata, capers and parsley	Spicy vegetable soup with red kidney beans and coriander
Snack	Fresh vegetable snack Serve of cheese	Serve of cheese Serve of nuts	Serve of fruit	Serve of cheese	Salmon muffins	Tofu balls with tamarind and tomato sauce	Serve of fruit
Dinner	Salmon muffins Simple rocket	Barbecued fish fillets	Chicken soup	Middle Eastern burgers	Vegetable salad Tomato salsa	Barbecued lamb cutlets Barbecued	Cajun beef stir-fry

One who knows their opponent and knows themselves will not be in danger in a hundred battles.

One who does not know their opponent but knows themselves will sometimes win, sometimes lose.

One who does not know their opponent and does not know themselves will be in danger in every battle.

Sun Tze 500 BC

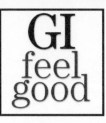

GI
feel
good

Health & weight loss

John Ratcliffe Dip. TCM, Grad Dip Psy

HINKLER
BOOKS

GI Feel Good: Health and Weight Loss
Published in 2005 by Hinkler Books Pty Ltd
17–23 Redwood Drive
Dingley VIC 3172 Australia
www.hinklerbooks.com

ISBN 1 7412 1899 3

Cover design: Sam Grimmer
Typesetting: Midland Typesetters
Printed and bound in Australia

This book is intended as a reference guide only. The information presented here is
designed to help you make informed choices about your health. It is not intended
as a substitute for any treatment or weight loss program prescribed by your
doctor.

Contents

Acknowledgments

I would like to thank my partner Chérie Van Styn who has tirelessly continued to come up with new recipes and moral support for the new book. Her selfless devotion and boundless energy to the task at hand has been a constant source of inspiration.

I would also like to thank Karin Serry, who is not only a great friend but was also the first person to draw my attention to GI.

And finally, to the many patients who took my advice and followed this way of eating, lost lots of weight, and had to buy new clothes.

TOLD YOU SO!

Carbohydrate: Carbohydrates are mainly vegetables, beans, legumes, grains and pulses, but things that come from vegetables (like starch and sugar) are also carbohydrates. If you were to think of carbs as sugars and sugar as carbs it would make the rest of the book easier to follow.

Protein: Meats like fish, chicken, lamb, beef and pork are protein.

Fats: Fats or lipids are concentrated energy that has been made into storage by something else. They include oils, butter and cheese.

Blood sugar levels: The amount of glucose in the blood.

Insulin: The hormone that controls the blood sugar levels.

Introduction

Welcome to *GI Feel Good: Health and Weight Loss.* By now, you have probably already heard about low carb and even the Glycemic Index (GI). It may seem like the latest thing but it may surprise you to know that low carb has been around since the 1960s and the GI since the end of the 1970s. My partner, Chérie Van Styn, and myself have released a number of books over the years on the subject of low carb and how to use GI and this is actually our fifth book.

The GI has made the biggest change to our thoughts about nutrition in over 30 years. Many years ago, when I first began researching the GI and low carb, the term 'low carb' always meant using carbohydrates with your meals that have a low GI, rather than restricting the intake of carbohydrates. The reason why I mention this is because many people are still confused and think it's about cutting all their carbs out of the diet. This is incorrect.

So, what is the GI and why is it different? Firstly, the GI helps you gauge the effect that carbohydrates will have on your blood sugar levels when you eat them. Why should that matter? Because understanding this allows you to control whether or not you will end up having lots of insulin in your blood. You see, when it comes to controlling your weight and looking after your health, insulin plays a major role.

Insulin is a very important hormone and it does many things in the body. Using 'low GI' carbs limits the action of insulin and as a result, among other things, we can eat quite well and control our weight and cholesterol at the same time. Now it shouldn't take too long before you realise that controlling your blood sugar levels and cholesterol is going to have a significant impact on such diseases as diabetes and heart disease, but what you may not know is that it also has a big impact on a number of other problems, in particular a major cause of infertility in women, called polycystic ovarian syndrome (PCOS).

When I began my training back in the 1980s, I never envisaged becoming an author; just understanding Traditional Chinese Medicine (TCM) was challenging enough. I spent a total of nine years studying TCM and have been treating patients for my entire adult life. Part of my study included three-and-a-half years of western medicine. Whilst we're on the subject I also spent two years doing a post-graduate in psychotherapy, Cognitive Behavioural Therapy (CBT) and the treatment of depression being my strong suit.

My interest in GI started in 1995. In those days the GI was barely a blip on the radar. When I first learnt about the GI, I pretty much knew that it was going to turn everything we thought on its head. Including fat in the diet? Not counting calories? Eating as much as you want? This was nutritional heresy. Posters with food pyramids adorned many doctors' waiting rooms and school canteens. The high wizards of nutrition had decreed for more than 30 years that 'Fat was the enemy' and we must do our utmost to rout it out. The World Health Organization (WHO) had for decades repeated the same ineffectual message of 'Eat a balanced diet', and then there was that one about 'Getting out there and do some work, you lazy good for nothing . . .'? Hang on a sec, I think that was my mother! Anyway you get the idea.

In spite of all this, society's waistline continued to expand. Could it be that we had yet to reach the high water mark of conventional wisdom about nutrition? Was there some hope on the horizon . . . a breakthrough?

Well that breakthrough came for me unexpectedly, when one of my patients, who had heard about the GI, asked me to look into this 'blood sugar thing'. She couldn't understand it but she felt that I would and may be I could explain it. This guided me to the work of Rick Mendosa. Rick, a medical journalist, had started to compile a resource website for diabetics. It was from this that I first started to understand the GI. As it turned out the research into the actual effect on blood sugar levels began in the late 70s–early 80s. That was 15 years earlier and I was just starting to learn about it now? Just think about it a moment, how long has it taken for this information to finally reach you? Believe it or not, there are many examples of this in medicine, but I digress.

Elements of the scientific community, particularly in the US, were trying to develop a more accurate way of helping diabetics with their diets. They were looking beyond the conventional wisdom of telling people to eat more complex carbohydrates like bread, pasta and grains and avoid simple carbohydrates like sugar, sweets and so on. Unfortunately this advice wasn't really getting to the bottom of what to eat. So a more enlightened approach was required. This came in a very simple and, in retrospect, obvious answer to the conundrum.

Diabetics are really good at measuring their blood sugar levels because it has to be done regularly throughout the day. Someone in the diabetics association came up with the idea of simply eating a range of carbohydrates and then measuring the blood sugar levels (BSLs) at different intervals and actually seeing what the carbohydrates were doing. They gave it a whirl and to their surprise, a lot of the carbohydrates they were told would have little effect on the blood sugar levels were doing the exact opposite. Instead of seeing a slow rise in the BSLs, some carbohydrates caused a dramatic increase. In some instances, the carbohydrate was behaving worse than sugar. After testing a wide range of carbohydrates, all of a sudden they were starting to get a handle on controlling the BSLs and insulin with their food. Out of this, the glycemic index was created. Now at the time these nice people weren't trying to save the world but their discovery was to have far-reaching consequences. Let us take a look at the GI and see how exactly it is worked out.

You take glucose and you give it to a number of people and then measure the effect it has on their BSLs. The rise is given as an 'index' of 100, just for something to compare the other things to. Then you take a carbohydrate, let the people eat it and retest the BSLs, comparing the rise in their BSLs to the glucose, and there you have the GI. Sounds simple enough?

For example, if people are given white bread, the rise in the BSLs from the bread is compared to the rise in BSLs when eating glucose. Glucose always has an arbitrary value of 100 because when the body breaks down carbohydrate, it always ends up as glucose in the blood, so that's what we use for comparison. We discover the bread has a GI of 90. So we could say that white bread affects the BSLs almost the same way glucose does.

Now this may all be well and good, but 'How is the GI going to help me?' I hear you ask. Fortunately the next chapter in the book is devoted entirely to explaining this, so I'm not going to spoil it. Back to the story.

So there I was, starting to come to grips with the idea that there was a way of controlling insulin via the GI. I soon realised that this would have a very big impact on controlling the way the body does things, in particular how it stores fat. I started experimenting with different food combinations to see how true it was and how it would affect one's weight. At the time, I was trying to 'eat healthily', and look after my weight with exercise, but those extra kilograms seemed very difficult to budge. After a few short months of playing around with the GI, not only had I lost the extra weight, I was the same weight I was when I was 18 years of age and although being (coughs) a fraction older, I was very pleased with the results.

Encouraged by this I began introducing the knowledge to my patients who eagerly wished to share the excitement. Before long I was receiving a steady stream of people coming to sit in my office for the hour or so it took for me to explain about the GI and how to use it. I had arranged a four-page summary on what we had discussed, so the people could take away some notes and for a couple of years this was sufficient. Every so often I would have a visit from someone I had met earlier, who just had to come back and show me the results. This actually became a weekly occurrence and I'll never forget one young lady who decided to strip down to her underwear, just so I could get a better impression. It's a little hard explaining to your beloved why a young woman is parading around your office in her underwear and you're not making any effort to avert your eyes!

Eventually, sitting and explaining the same lesson over and over started taking its toll, so I contemplated writing it all down in a book that I might just give to my patients instead. So writing on the subject began in earnest and after about nine months I was putting the finishing touches on my first book *Sugar Science*. It covered the basics and included about 50 recipes that Chérie had put together, as examples of the types of meals that one included in a low GI diet.

Getting a book printed and bound in small numbers is a costly exercise, but before long we were eagerly tearing open the box of the first 500 spiral-bound copies. So instead of me having to explain it in person, I could just hand a book to the patient and they could read about it. Before long, we were selling out and even a big city bookstore had started to stock our humble book for its customers.

By now I was starting to realise that the GI was developing momentum. I had told a few thousand people, and the vast majority all had good results. I rationalised that thousands more would probably get the same results and so hundreds of thousands would probably benefit from the same knowledge and so on and so on. So I stayed the course, kept releasing more books and Chérie kept coming up with new recipes, right up to the present-day where we come to *GI Feel Good: Health and Weight Loss*, the latest addition to our collection of books.

Over the years I have personally witnessed many people do well by following our books. The popularity of the original book was spread purely from one person telling another and this continues to the present day. There's a good bet you are reading this because someone you know has told you to read it. See what I mean? But enough about me and the book. This brings us to the part where you can now go on to learn the mechanics of the GI and how to use the knowledge.

Explaining how to use the GI is actually very, very easy. Explaining the science behind it, however, is extremely complicated. Please be aware that I have left out a lot of complex explanations to try to make it as easy and as simple as possible for you to follow. When you have finished reading the book, you should have a very effective way of dealing with your health and in particular your weight. Coincidentally, why did I concentrate on the weight loss side of things? Because controlling your weight has a flow-on effects on many other health issues. If you can look after your weight then you can control many other things, like heart disease, diabetes and so on.

GI Feel Good: Health and Weight Loss is a formula that we have refined and developed over almost a decade and although this may seem like a long time, we are still tweaking and tuning it every so often to try to make it better. I believe that we have developed a way of using the glycemic index that is extremely effective at achieving its objectives. There are some great books on the GI, but by and large they fail to focus on weight and health issues, but rather provide general information. You will find that where we draw the line on what is a good carb, and what isn't, is slightly lower than other books. Sometimes it's mostly from practise but also we try to keep it that way to ensure that you can achieve your desired outcome with as little effort as possible. The science behind a lot of what I write can be found in any good physiology book, but what is also here is the experience of helping thousands of people individually, one-on-one, follow a low GI diet.

Read the book thoroughly and try not to skip sections. Everything you need to know is in this book and then some. Make yourself familiar with the information and get used to the concepts even if it may seem counterintuitive to your conventional thinking and always remember we have a fantastic website (www.glycemic-index.com) that can be a great source of support and information any time you may have questions. After you have read the book and have put the principles into practice, you, dear reader, can be the judge and decide for yourself the benefits of understanding the GI. Don't be surprised if you find that this exciting knowledge changes your life. You may even end up like the rest of us, still using the GI after many years, quite happy with your choices and the on-going benefits gained.

CHAPTER 1

What's it all about?

The story so far

Nutrition may be a very important topic to you and I, but is a poor cousin twice removed when it comes to medical science. Medicine has streaked away with research dollars discovering all sorts of things. Nutrition, on the other hand, holds little monetary value by comparison, in spite of the fact that what we eat has the biggest impact on our health.

In recent years we have seen the sequencing of the human genome, stem cell therapy, the bionic ear and so on. By comparison, as far as nutrition goes, the most significant discovery in the past century occurred around the time of the Second World War and, as usual, by accident. Two fellows in white coats were having a slow morning at the research lab, when one decided that setting the other's morning tea alight was going to be worth a giggle. Unfortunately in the process of the prank, he was caught by his supervisor. The quick-thinking scientist explained that he was just trying to see how much heat his friend's doughnut gave off. 'Great stuff', replied the supervisor, 'Have the full report on my desk by Friday.' Whether you like my version or not, this was more or less how calories were discovered. Now everyone has heard about calories, and just about every diet that you care to name owes its origin to this experiment and the pyromaniac who thought of it. In essence, calories are worked out by placing a certain amount of food, or the carbohydrate that the food contains, over a Bunsen burner and setting it alight. A beaker of water is placed over the burning food and for every degree that the temperature in the beaker rises, it is multiplied by one hundred – this gives you the calories of that food. So if something is 300 calories, it caused the water temperature to rise by three degrees. It may come as a surprise to some that such an abstract way of determining the amount of energy food contains has become so well-known. The reason of course is it's a sound theory.

The body needs energy to survive and it gets its energy from the food that we eat and, in particular, from the carbo-hydrates. If we can work out how much energy we are giving the body, then we can get a handle on how much we should have before we start over-feeding ourselves. So the basic premises is, if the amount of energy in the diet is less that the output of energy from the person, then there is a deficit and the person must lose weight. This is correct and there are many low calorie diets around that, providing people stick to them, cause people to lose weight. These diets generally use very little or no fat and require you to exercise. The reason behind this, if you haven't already worked it out, is by doing exercise you increase your energy output. Doing exercise and keeping energy input to a minimum, the body has to lose weight. Eating less fat, which is a very high source of energy, helps quite a lot. Anyone who has ever seen sausages burn on a BBQ, and if you have lived in Australia then who hasn't, will remember great flames leaping about. Why? That's the energy in the fat being oxidised (burnt) along with the hair on your host's forearms and eyebrows.

We know from experience that low calorie diets help people to lose weight and that cutting out fat is very important. Even though there seems to be thousands of different types of diets, they all, in one way or another, come down to the same thing: less calories means less weight. But the funny thing is we have been cutting fat out of our diets for almost 30 years. Many experts are questioning whether or not this strategy is really working. Surely since the 1940s we must have learnt something else about food? For many the GI is the next step forward. To understand this we need to understand how the body absorbs its energy.

There's only one tiny problem with low calorie diets. Remember how calories are worked out by setting food on fire? This is where we get this idea about the body 'burning up energy' and so forth. Funnily enough, when we eat, have you ever noticed how the food never actually bursts into flames? Even after you have eaten, have you ever wondered why there seems to be a distinct lack of smoke and fire as you digest?

The reason for this is because the way the body extracts the energy from the food is far more sophisticated and complex than this. In fact some of the steps in the process are so involved they are still theoretical. But this doesn't mean you can't understand it, in fact I can explain the basics quite easily. If we were to distil the way the body absorbs energy down to its lowest common denominator, we could isolate it to the action of a single hormone. That hormone would be insulin.

Insulin and carbohydrates

When we eat a meal, almost without exception, we will include carbohydrates. It's the bread roll that's wrapped around the salad you had for lunch, it's the two or three potatoes on the side of your plate when you're having a roast, the flour used to thicken the sauce or even the sugar that someone has added to your food to make it taste nicer. You see the body wants energy and it gets its energy from carbohydrates. When we eat something that has carbohydrates the body happily breaks it down to glucose to get what it needs.

How much would that be? Well the average person has about 5 grams of glucose in their blood at any one time. That's roughly a heaped teaspoon. Not a lot. What's left over gets converted into a gooey syrup called glycogen (gly-co-gen), which is stored in the liver and muscle for later use. The body can convert the glycogen back into glucose and re-release it if the glucose levels fall, but there is only a limited amount that can be put away. The body stores about 500 ml (2 cups) of glycogen and when it has enough it then does a very peculiar thing: the remaining glycogen goes on to be converted into fat.

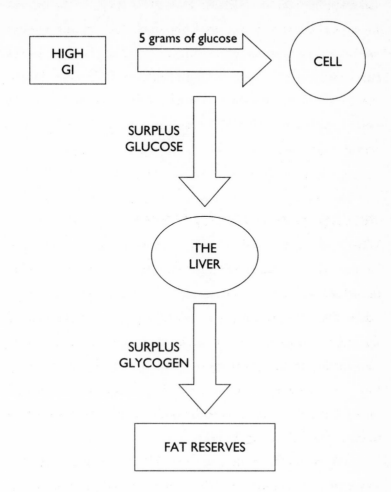

What this effectively means is you can eat carbohy-drates that contain no fat whatsoever, but a certain percentage of what you are eating will be turned into fat by the body. That is why eating something that is '99% fat-free' can still be fattening and why people who have a low-fat diet can still have a cholesterol problem as well as a weight problem. But before you start throwing out all the so-called 'healthy' food in your pantry, there's the other bit about fats contained in the diet.

Dietary fat and carbohydrate

When you eat something that contains fat, fat on its own does not raise your blood sugar levels. For your body to store it, the blood sugar levels have to be raised and insulin released. What raises your blood sugar levels? Carbohydrates with a moderate-to-high GI. The funny thing is we intuitively add carbs to fats so we can absorb it, like the examples I gave before: the bread with the butter, the potato with the roast and so on. The reason for this is because without the carbohydrate there will be no insulin and without insulin the fat doesn't get pushed into the adipose tissue, the fat cells where it normally gets stored. So take, for example, something like bacon and eggs. It contains fat and protein but no carbohydrate – even though you are thinking you're absorbing the fat in actual fact your body cannot store it without the carbohydrate and eventually the fat passes back out of the body several hours later. Something else you will discover is why you actually would lose weight from this, but more about that later. If you instead added something that had a moderate-to-high GI, like bread or beans, then the whole thing takes on a different perspective: insulin would be released and the fat would be allowed to go into storage.

So essentially it's about insulin and the blood sugar levels. Blood sugar levels are influenced by carbohydrate (glucose) and insulin is influenced by blood sugar levels. If there is a way of controlling the blood sugar levels, then we have a way to control insulin and, as a result, control what our body does with all the surplus energy we throw at it. Put another way, imagine if there was a way we could still eat yummy food but cleverly avoid any of it becoming storage.

Even better, what if we could eat yummy food and actually make our bodies give up the fat that it had in storage and lose weight at the same time . . .! Enter the glycemic index.

The glycemic index

The glycemic index has always been about insulin. Remember when the diabetic's association started the first experiments? A group of people eating different types of carbohydrates, measuring their blood sugar levels and comparing with glucose? They were trying to discover which carbohydrates didn't cause insulin to be released. To understand this we have to look more closely at how insulin works.

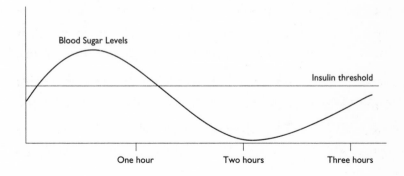

You may have seen a graph like this before, showing you how the rise in the blood sugar levels past a certain point causes insulin to be released. When insulin is released and the blood sugar levels start to fall, what is actually happening is the body has started converting the excess sugars into glycogen and eventually fat. That has been the way the body has dealt with excess blood sugar levels since the time of creation.

So what the GI told us was that some carbohydrates were just like glucose and caused insulin to be released, some were just on the borderline and some were so low it didn't matter how much one ate, it would never be enough to raise the BSLs. If we put that into a table it would look something like the one on page 25. I must warn you if this is the first time you have seen the GI, make sure you are sitting down.

Using the glycemic index

Quite often, when doing an interview, the first question I am asked is 'So why are carbohydrates bad'? I always answer that it's the context which matters. If we think of carbo-hydrate in terms of nourishment, then *all* carbohydrates are good. However if we are trying to control our weight, lower our cholesterol, prevent diabetes, prevent heart disease and, in the case of a woman, become fertile, then in this context there are many carbohydrates that can be considered bad. In this context, we have three tables: the high GI or 'bad carbs', medium GI or 'good carbs' and the low GI 'excellent carbs'. But how can we use this knowledge for our health?

The liver as a fuel tank

Earlier I mentioned that the liver stores glycogen, and the body uses the glycogen as a source of fuel when the glucose levels fall. When only eating moderate and low GI carbohydrates, the body is not getting a surplus of glucose. This means that although these carbohydrates still give us energy, they are insufficient to add to the storage that we have in the liver. If

The GI of certain carbohydrates

Maltose	110
Glucose	**100**
Parsnips	97
White bread	90
White rice	87
Potato	**85**
Honey	75
Pumpkin	75
Sugar	**72**
Pasta	70
Carrots	70
Cornflakes	70
Popcorn	70
Chocolate bar	70
Corn	70
Beetroot	65
Banana	60
Jam	55
Spaghetti	55
Whole rye bread	50
Fresh pasta	40
Beans	30
Lentils	30
Fresh fruit	30
Fructose	20
Lettuce, tomato, mushroom	15

we keep using these carbs, the glycogen stored in the liver gradually begins to be used up. Whilst this is happening, you still feel like you have plenty of energy because the body is making up to any differences by using its reserves to maintain the glucose levels in your blood. For most people it takes about three days for all the glycogen to get used up. Now here comes the exciting bit. After the glycogen runs out, the body does a very unusual thing. It starts using the fat for fuel.

What the body is doing here is converting the fat back into what it started off as originally, namely glucose. When the body is using the fat for fuel, guess what? We begin to gradually lose weight. As long as the liver is empty of glycogen the weight loss continues, and it is important to stay away from things that will create a surplus of glucose like the high GI carbs.

Now you understand how following GI works. Quite simple isn't it? Next is the lowdown on how to use this knowledge to achieve results.

Using the GI for health and weight loss

Moderate GI carbs

To make it happen, naturally the high GI carbs are off the menu. Not only do they stop you from losing weight but they can also make you put on weight. This leaves us with the medium GI carbs and the low GI carbs. When it comes to whether or not you will produce any insulin when you eat them, the medium GI carbs are typically close to the border-

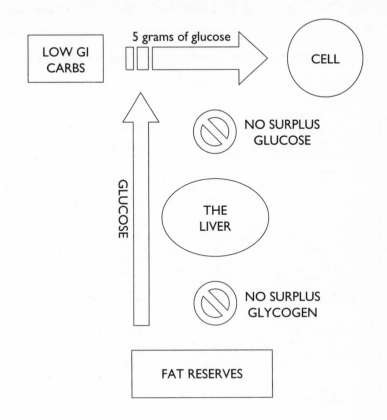

line. Because these carbohydrates generally will not produce enough glucose to create a surplus then there is no concern about putting on weight when we use them. However we assume that there may be an insulin response, and because having insulin around will give our bodies an opportunity to absorb any fats in the meal, what we do is avoid adding any fats or oils, butter, meats and cheeses to this meal when we eat them. If we can't add any fats, oils, butter, meats or cheeses, then what else can we have with them?

The low GI carbs of course. So what you end up with is a meal of moderate and low GI carbohydrates, without oil, butter, meats or cheeses: in other words a vegetarian dish, like a risotto or pasta Napoli and the selection of food would look something like this.

Moderate carbs	Good carbs
Whole cereals	Alfalfa sprouts
Wheat, oats,	Celery
Barley, millet	Bamboo shoots
Bran	Cucumber
Pure rye	Tomato
Bread*	Radish
Basmati rice*	Lettuce
Fresh pasta*	Cauliflower
Vermicelli*	Broccoli
Wheatgerm	Eggplant
Dried beans	Mushroom
Lentils	Cabbage
Sweet potato	Artichokes
Yams	Peppers
Soy beans	Spinach
Chickpeas	Squash
Fresh and dried fruit*	
*These are exceptions which are explained later	

From the table we can see that by combining what is on the moderate carb list with those in the good carb list basically results in our choices for the meal. This type of meal from now on we shall refer to as the *carbohydrate meal*. It may also get referred to as the 'carb meal' for short. All the rules that apply to moderate carbohydrates applies to this meal.

Protein meals

The second type of meals is when we leave out the moderate carbs and only use the low GI carbs. When we do this there is no risk whatsoever of raising blood sugar levels because the GI of these type of carbohydrates are very low. We can now include the meats, cheeses, butters and oils because these things will not affect the blood sugar levels either and, as a result, no insulin, and no fat, gets stored. So if you want to have rack of lamb with vegetables like broccoli, zucchini and/or eggplant, you can. In winter, one of my favourites is roast squash and asparagus with a cheese sauce and a roast, and probably barbecue lamb and a green salad with tomato and cucumber in the summer. When we introduce the meats, fish, poultry, oils, fats, eggs and cheeses in combination with the low GI carbs, the choice of food would look something like the following table on page 30.

This type of meal is more the 'business end' of low GI and we refer to this type of meal as the *protein meal*.

You now have two types of meals: one which raises your blood sugar levels slightly, but does not contain any fats and another that contains fats but does not affect your blood sugar levels. That is basically the nuts and bolts of the GI, but before you fire up the BBQ and start charcoaling that slab of cow in the freezer, there are a few other things you need to be aware of.

Good carbs	Proteins, fats and oils
Alfalfa sprouts	Meats
Celery	Poultry
Bamboo shoots	Lamb
Cucumber	Pork
Tomato	Ham
Radish	Beef
Lettuce	Veal
Cauliflower	Rabbit
Broccoli	Kangaroo
Eggplant	Eggs
Mushroom	Fish
Cabbage	Lobster
Artichokes	Crab
Peppers	Prawns/shrimp
Spinach	Butter
Squash	Margarine
	Cheese
	Oils

Time windows

When we use the GI, generally we don't just eat one type of meal exclusively, say, for example, eating carb meals only or protein meals only. Instead we swap from one meal type to another through the day, like carbohydrate meal for breakfast and protein lunch and so on. When we do this it adds another consideration.

When you eat a carb meal, you will get a rise in BSLs, which is not a problem because you are not creating a surplus of glucose and should not affect your weight loss. However, having a little bit of insulin floating around in your blood does make it possible for you to absorb any fats in the meal. So at this stage we have to be very careful about including fats with the meal. The funny part is it takes about three hours for your blood sugar levels to normalise again. During this time you cannot eat any fats or cheeses because the little bit of insulin would allow the body to absorb those fats. So here is the first rule when eating carb meals:

> When eating moderate carb meals you must wait at least three hours before having a protein meal.

The protein meal

When you eat a protein meal, although it has no effect on the BSLs, you will still be able to absorb the fat for up to *five hours* afterwards if you raise your blood sugar levels. The reason for this is because the duodenum is where the body absorbs fat from. It lies immediately after the stomach and it takes about five hours for the meal to pass through this area before it passes into the small intestine where other nutrients are absorbed. If you ate any moderate carbs after you had your protein meal, you will raise your blood sugar levels and give the insulin an opportunity to absorb the fat. This is highly undesirable, so you need to wait five hours for the fats to pass out of the duodenum, before eating moderate carbs again. Therefore:

31

> When eating a protein meal or anything that contains fats you must wait at least five hours before eating moderate carbs.

If your head is starting to swim and you're feeling confused right now, don't worry, this is the only thinking bit you are going to come across. If you are able to understand this, congratulations, you're passing with flying colours. Stand up and read aloud so that everyone can hear you – no hang on a sec maybe that's not such a good idea. Better to read more just so you fully understand. Try reading quietly to yourself for now, if you're having trouble. This next bit should help.

> These time intervals only apply if you are swapping from a carb meal to a protein meal or a protein meal to a carb meal.

So how does this play itself out in the real world? If, for example, like most people you like to eat a carb breakfast like muesli and then are planning to have a protein meal like chicken breast and salad for lunch, you have to be sure that breakfast was before 9 am if lunch is at 12 pm: in other words a three-hour wait for the BSLs to normalise before eating anything that may contain fat like the chicken. Vice versa if you happened to have lamb and vegetables for lunch and were planning on having pasta for dinner: you would have to wait five hours after lunch before eating the pasta. So if lunch finished about 1 pm then you would have to wait until 6 pm before having the pasta.

If you have a carb breakfast and a protein lunch and then planned for protein again for dinner, would you have to wait? Between breakfast and lunch, yes, you would wait three hours, but is there any need to wait again before eating after lunch? No, because you are not swapping back to carbs again. Because lunch and dinner are both protein meals then there is no need to wait. If you wanted to have dinner earlier it would make no difference. The time windows *only apply when you swap* from one type of meal to another. *Carb to protein three hours and protein to carb five hours.* So now its time for the pop quiz.

Caution: humour ahead

Question 1: You have had your carb breakfast at 7.30 am and now it's 10 am and you're getting a little peckish and you decide to eat some fruit, another moderate carb. Which of the following is correct?

> A. You extend the time window by another three hours and must wait another three hours before eating anything that contains fat.
>
> B. The carb breakfast was almost three hours ago, eating fruit now will not make any difference.
>
> C. What's a carbohydrate?

The answer is A. If you were planning on eating a protein meal for lunch then you would have to put that off until after one pm. Alternatively you could just find yourself another carb meal for lunch.

Question 2: On another day you have had a beautiful piece of grilled fish and salad for lunch. A couple of hours later someone offers you a mandarin. Do you:

A. Start eating the mandarin, completely unaware that all the fat from lunch is now being absorbed?

B. Start eating the mandarin and then suddenly spit it out, look confused and run from the room?

C. Take the mandarin from your friend, place it on the floor and squash it with your foot before walking off?

D. Politely take the mandarin, saying 'I'll save this for later,' wait five hours and then eat it?

E. Politely refuse and explain you'll be eating some cheese instead?

If you answered D and E, you would be correct. If you answered any of the others, you would have been mistaken and possibly have sociopathic tendencies . . .

Question 3: You have had a protein lunch and are feeling a little peckish at around five pm. You are planning on having another protein meal for dinner in a couple of hours and you would like a snack now. Do you:

A. Fight your hunger and wait patiently for dinner.

B. Find something that is also protein, like cheese or sliced ham and eat that?

C. Find something that has the low GI, like celery, tomato, alfalfa and eat that?

D. Find something that has the low GI like celery, tomato, alfalfa and eat that with the cheese or the ham?

E. Find your friend with the mandarin and beg them to give you another chance?

A, B, C and D would all be correct. If you answered E then

perhaps read this section over again. Eating moderate carbs will raise your blood sugar levels so by the time you sat down to dinner two hours later, your blood sugar levels may still be elevated and any fats contained in the meal would be absorbed.

If you think you have the hang of this, then very good. The time windows are the only thing that requires any real thinking, the rest is pretty easy so you're off to a great start. What follows are just a few extra rules that you need to follow.

The exceptions

Milk: Cow's milk is lactose, and lactose is a sugar. Milk has a moderate GI but, from experience, we have found that lactose seems to effect the glycogen levels and holds up the results. So we recommend you make the switch from cow's milk to soymilk. Now you may have tried soymilk and reached the conclusion that it tastes fairly average and I would agree, having tried a great many brands. Before you start your own process, the type of soymilk you use shouldn't contain sugar or malt. The brand we use is 'Australia's Own Malt-Free soy milk' which, I must say, I enjoy the taste of but will admit it is probably an acquired one. (Funnily enough, it's the taste of milk that I can't stand now.) Australia's Own Malt-Free is available in most supermarkets – look in the health food section. If you can't get your hands on it then another alternative is the brand called Soy King. It is slightly more expensive and not quite the same in taste but it will do as an alternative. If you live somewhere else and can't get these brands then the one with the lowest sugar per 100ml should be your choice. To give you an idea Australia's Own Malt-Free is 0.4g per 100ml.

As far as cow's milk goes there are many varieties with a moderate GI. You are quite welcome to experiment with cow's milk if you like but from our experience it can negate the effect of following GI and we don't advise it. So if you want to get the best results then perhaps now is the time to get use to drinking soymilk.

Caffeine: Caffeine unfortunately causes insulin to be released, so things that contain caffeine, like tea and coffee, can't be included with your protein meals because the insulin will cause the fat in the meal to be absorbed. The good news is you can have them with carb meals, so if you are one of those people who can't get going without a coffee in the morning then with your carb breakfast it's ok. Obviously no sugar, cow juice or cream. You can put soymilk in coffee, you just have to add it first and slowly pour in the water.

If you wanted to have a hot drink with the protein meal then decaf is the way to proceed. We have always used a low caffeine tea called Madura tea – it tastes like black tea and we have it with everything. If you can't get it, don't panic – most teas are low caffeine. Buy the brand which tells you the amount – Madura tea is 3% for example. I myself seldom drink coffee. Decaf coffee is okay, the reason I never drink decaf is because the way they get the caffeine out of the coffee requires certain chemicals that aren't very good for your health, so I prefer Madura tea instead. Herbal teas are also fine, just be careful with some of the fruit teas, as they can be a little sweet on the palate.

Bread: There are only a handful of breads that have a GI lower then 50; all the rest are so high you may as well be eating cake. Some of the breads with a GI lower than 50 contain fat, which rules them out as well. These include the soy and linseed breads and the honey and oat bran breads. If you want to eat them, you have to be aware of the fat content. The fats will be going on your waistline, which is not the idea. That's the bad news: the good news is a type of bread that we know of that has a low GI and does not contain fat, and that is bread made from triticale. Triticale is a hybrid rye/wheat. Don't worry, it's not genetically modified; triticale has been around for ages and you end up with a loaf that looks like brown bread. The brand is called 'Performax' and the makers are 'Country Life Bakeries'. You should be able to find it in most supermarkets. 'Performax' has a GI of 38 and is a moderate carb.

Fruit: If you regard fruit as a moderate carb you shouldn't have any problems and, as with all moderate carbs, eat them in moderation. The sugar contained in fruit is *fructose* and, although it tastes sweet, it doesn't seem to have the same impact on the blood sugar levels as normal sugar does. But that doesn't mean going overboard and eating big bowls of fruit in an attempt to make up for the lack of sugar in the diet, it will bring you unstuck. There are a few fruits that do cross the line; they are *banana, grapes, cantaloupe* and *watermelon.* So these have to be excluded.

The other thing that you need to watch out for is juices. An apple, for example, may have a moderate GI but if you extract the juice from the apple you are getting rid of the flesh and you are concentrating the sugars, making it easier for the body to absorb. This will raise the GI slightly and from the tables at the back of the book you can see that the GI of apple juice is higher than an apple. That's not to say avoid drinking juice, it's just something that you need to be mindful of and if you start having trouble getting the weight down this is something you may need to re-examine.

Fresh pasta versus dried pasta: Fresh pasta is a moderate GI carb but dried pasta is a high GI carb, so what's the story here?

The reason is that any pasta that takes more than five minutes to cook is going to have a high GI. This is because the heat from cooking causes the carbohydrates in the pasta to swell and increase their surface area. If something has a larger surface area it means there is more of it in touch with the outside world, meaning the body can absorb more carbohydrate easier.

Let me put it another way. Try to imagine at a microscopic level that the carbohydrates in the pasta look like tennis balls before you cook them, and when you heat them they start to expand, so that after ten minutes they have totally expanded to the size of basketballs. The less time it takes to cook, the less they expand. Do you know the old trick of throwing the pasta against the wall to see if it is cooked? It's cooked because it's the expanded sugar that makes it stick to the wall.

Where I come from, fresh pasta is usually fettuccine. You either make it yourself, or buy it at a deli or supermarket, and it is one of the few types of pasta that is cooked in less than five minutes, but here's where you need to be careful. *Don't overcook the pasta.* If it is still not cooked after five minutes, it is not the right kind.

Basmati rice versus brown and white rice: Many people regard rice as health food and for most of Asia it is. But when it comes to trying to keep control of your blood sugar levels, brown and white rices' GI is very similar to sugar. Fortunately there is a type of rice that originated in India called basmati rice. It has a moderate GI. When you go to an Indian restaurant, have you ever noticed how the rice they serve is fluffy? That's because it's basmati rice; it doesn't stick together because it has less glucose in it than normal rice. This rice has carbohydrate polymers that are different to other rice. On a microscopic level, normal rice carbohydrates are chains that are strung together with many branches, like a pine frond, giving them a greater surface area. Basmati rice is more like a single chain – as a result less glucose and less stickiness. 'Mahatma Premium' is a popular brand in Australia. There is another type of rice that is also available; the name is 'Doongara'. You should also be able to find this in the local supermarket.

Eating moderate carbs in moderation

Moderate carbs meals have more energy as far as the carbo-hydrate goes when compared to the protein meals. When eating moderate carbohydrate meals, we have found that it is best to be moderate because eating too much of the moderate carbs can gradually restore the glycogen in the liver and hold up your progress. Now this can vary from person to person and you will need to find your own balance here. I person-ally have carbs for breakfast and usually protein for lunch and dinner. Occasionally I will include a carb lunch/dinner here and there and I find this works best for me. Chérie, on the other hand, can eat carbs all day and it doesn't seem to make any difference. Other people are different but the golden rule with moderate carbs is to eat them in modera-tion. Originally I used to tell people that they can eat as much as they like. Why? Because for many years it never caused a problem but eventually people turned up who were still having trouble losing weight. What I discovered was they were eating huge bowls of fruit in the morning or pasta or several slices of bread and this was undoing all their good work. The reason why they did this was simply to compensate for the lack of sugar in the diet, so they made up for it by eating as much of the moderate carbohydrates as they could. Don't make this mistake, it will make you unhappy. So we have one last rule:

Be moderate with the moderate carbohydrates.

So it's time for you to relax and embark on the great adventure and discover why the GI is making the biggest impact on the way we think about food in over fifty years.

Next in this book are the recipes and the meal planner. Prepare yourself to be amazed by what you can eat!

Chérie will take it from here and guide you through this section herself.

21–day
meal planner

and

recipes

21-day meal planner

About the meal planner

Shopping and cooking tips A to Z

Day 0 to 21 menus, instructions, shopping and cooking

Finishing the meal planner

About the meal planner

The 21-day meal planner is designed to get you started on the *GI Feel Good: Health and Weight Loss* plan. It is designed for two people working Monday to Friday, but you can alter it to suit the number of people you are feeding and your time schedule. The planner allows you to eat interesting, tasty and varied food that will improve your health and help you to lose weight. The food is all low GI, nutritionally balanced, and follows the *GI Feel Good: Health and Weight Loss* formula. The meal planner guides you step-by-step through each meal in the week using simple and clear instructions, so that you will be successful following this style of eating.

The meal planner includes breakfasts, lunches, afternoon snacks and dinners, as well as instructions for meal preparation and planning for each day. All the recipes for the meal planner can be found in the recipe section by searching through the recipe index at the back of the book; you can even find the type of fruit and cheese you can eat, and what you should put on your cereal in the morning.

The meal planner also designates every Sunday and Wednesday as shopping and cooking days. A shopping list is written for each of these days every week, while lists of the food you will need to prepare in advance for the following days are also included. This way you will be more prepared with less time required for food preparation throughout your day. Plan to succeed by following all the preparation guides. Day 0 is your planning day; you should do all the suggested shopping and cooking on this day in preparation for starting the meal planner on Day 1. On Day 0 you should also throw out or give away all the bad carbohydrates from your pantry and refrigerator.

A wall planner has been included at the back of the book to give you an overview of all 21 days of the meal plan at a glance; stick it on your fridge. You will notice the wall planner is also colour-coded to make it easier for you to identify the meal types and following your time windows.

Remember to wait three hours after eating a carbohydrate meal before eating a protein meal, and wait five hours after eating a protein meal before eating a carbohydrate meal. Always eat moderate carbohydrates in moderation.

This plan is designed for a healthy adult. Children, teenagers, pregnant women and people with illnesses have different nutritional requirements and should consult their dietician or health professional. You should consult your health professional before beginning any dietary plan.

Shopping and cooking tips A to Z

GI Feel Good: Health and Weight Loss is a new approach to a healthy diet. You will find that shopping and cooking in this way is also new and different. You will become better at applying the *GI Feel Good: Health and Weight Loss* knowledge, cooking low GI food, and finding low GI ingredients in the supermarket over time. From my own experience I initially found cooking in this way to be a new and interesting challenge; of course, back then, there were no low GI recipe books to guide me through the taste experience that this way of eating offers. Now, however, I find this way of cooking the easiest, and I don't remember cooking any other way. Don't ask me how to cook potatoes now, I have completely forgotten!

Shopping for *GI Feel Good: Health and Weight Loss* ingredients is initially a steep learning curve, but persevere and you will become good at it; in fact it becomes time-saving because you no longer need to waste time in the lolly, chip, soft drink and biscuit aisles of the supermarket. Also reading the labels is a bit of an eye-opener if you have never had a good look at what you are really eating. You will be surprised by what actually goes into your food, particularly how much sugar.

I also try to use a wide variety of ingredients in my recipes so that you get a good range of interesting flavours, textures and nutrients in your diet. Don't be put off by ingredients you have not used before, believe me, they will eventually become a staple part of your culinary range. If you do not like some of the meals suggested in the meal planner, you are a vegetarian or you have allergies to some of the ingredients, then make your way to our website where you will find a great database of recipes to choose from. Our cookbooks also offer more recipes from which you can design your own meal plan.

The follow is a list of A–Z ingredients, cooking and shopping tips that you might find helpful for your new way of eating.

A All-bran

Even though many of the all-bran products in the supermarket seem to have added sugar, those that have been tested have been found to have a GI less than 50. It is safe to assume that moderate amounts of all-bran are suitable for moderate carbohydrate meals when following *GI Feel Good: Health and Weight Loss.*

Allergies

Some people may find they have a reaction to some of the food or ingredients suggested in the meal planner, such as shellfish, tomatoes and spicy food. Substitute ingredients using the *Healthy Shopper's Glycemic Index Pocket Guide* or find substitute recipes from our website www.glycemic-index.com or other cookbooks. We have lots of recipes – I am sure you will be able to find something to suit your needs.

Artificial sweeteners

You should avoid artificial sweeteners where possible. These include xylitol, maltitol, aspartame and litesse.

B	Bread	The brand of bread I use is 'Performax' by Country Life Bakeries. This bread has a GI less than 50 and contains minimal amounts of fat per serve. It is made from triticale. Some brands of bread may have a GI of less than 50. Look at the packet and read how much fat it contains. If it's only a few grams then why worry. If it's a lot then you have to keep looking. 'Performax' has 4.2g fat per 100g whereas another brand of soy and linseed has a GI of 36 but fat content of 7g per 100ml, which is a little too much. A teaspoon of fat is about 4g − 7g is almost double.
C	Canned beans	The brand I use is Annalisa. Generally all the canned beans with this brand do not have added sugar, however remember to always check the label. Read the section on sugar for more information on choosing brands.
	Cream	You should use cream, sour cream and mascarpone cheese in moderation. The small amount of lactose present in these products may cause weight loss to plateau for some people. Follow the amounts in the recipes and don't go

overboard adding extra cream here and there.

D	Dessert	Have fruit after carbohydrate meals and a cheese platter with protein meals if you feel the need to have dessert. People have experimented with artificially sweetened jellies and cheesecake and tablespoons of frozen cream; we suggest not to do this as it will cause your weight loss to plateau.
G	GI labelling	Beware of brands that claim their product has a low GI but don't have an actual GI figure written on their packaging. The Australian Competition and Consumer Commission (ACCC) has even taken some companies to task for falsely advertising that their products have a low GI when they do not. Products labelled with the GI symbol from Sydney University have all been properly tested.
	Goat's cheese	Goat's cheese has a higher lactose content than other types of cheese. For this reason we classify goat's cheese as a carbohydrate/lipid which should also be avoided.
H	Herbs	A lot of our recipes call for the use of fresh herbs. Fresh herbs

add flavour, particularly when you are no longer relying on sugar to flavour your meals. The best way to store fresh herbs is to keep them in a resealable plastic bag in the vegetable crisper of your refrigerator. Herbs generally last longer when stored at temperatures between 4.5–7°C. If it is too warm the herbs will wilt, whereas too cold and the leaves will blacken. Do not wash the herbs before storing, as the drier the leaves the longer they will keep. You can also freeze fresh herbs such as parsley by layering the leaves in a resealable plastic bag, then tightly rolling up the bag, securing with rubber bands, then placing in the freezer until required. In a pinch you may substitute fresh herbs with dried herbs – simply divide the required quantity of fresh herbs by three to calculate the required dried herbs for the recipe. For example, three tablespoons of fresh parsley could be substituted with one tablespoon of dried parsley.

K Kumara

Kumara is the New Zealand variety of sweet potato. Unfortunately Kumara has a GI above 50. However the Australian variety of sweet potato has a lower GI and is suitable for following the *GI Feel Good: Health and Weight Loss* plan.

O   Oil

Always use good quality olive oil when cooking, particularly in salads where it gives such a lovely flavour. If you wish to use other types of oils then vegetable and canola oils will work just as well. You may also use ghee and butter as a substitute for olive oil when stir-frying protein meals.

Onions

Onions are classified as a good carbohydrate. You can use them in both carbohydrate and protein meals, however you should not attempt to caramelise the onion as this changes its molecular structure and may cause a higher GI. When cooking onions for a carbohydrate meal you can either cook them in a non-stick frying pan with a little water, or place them in a microwave oven for one to two minutes or until softened.

P   Parmesan cheese

Some brands of parmesan cheese that you find pre-grated on the supermarket shelf actually have added rice flour and/or sugar. Always check the label when purchasing this product.

R	Recipes	All our recipes are created and written by me, the resident cook, Chérie Van Styn. There are hundreds of recipes that you can access through our website and our cookbooks. Read other GI enthusiasts' recipes on the website forum and submit your own.
S	Salt	If you are on a salt-restricted diet due to heart disease or other health problems then use less salt in your cooking. This means modifying the recipes in this book to decrease your salt intake.
	Shopper's Pocket Guide	The *Healthy Shopper's Glycemic Index Pocket Guide* is an excellent resource for identifying which products fit into which categories in the GI plan. It is broken into sections of bad carbohydrates, moderate carbohydrates, good carbohydrates, carbohydrate/lipids, proteins and unclassified foods. More and more food manufacturers are placing information about the glycemic index of their products on their packaging. You can keep updated with this new information and any new product innovations through our website.
	Stocks	All supermarket varieties have added sugar, so you will have to

make your own stock. There is a recipe for vegetable stock included in this book while recipes for fish, chicken and beef stock can be found on our website. Some people have tried using lightly salted water as a substitute for stock – you can try it if you like, it may work but I am not going to give any guarantees on the flavour.

Sugar

Sugar is added to products for preserving as well as for flavour. When checking products that do not have a known GI we usually reject them if they have added sugar. The added sugar may give the product a high GI. Other names for sugar that you should watch out for include maltose, maltodextrose, glucose, dextrose, lactose, sucrose and corn syrup. However some products have only very small amounts of sugar added and therefore may not cause our blood sugar levels to rise. Generally when deciding whether or not the sugar content is small enough to be harmless the following rule of thumb applies:

1. For products that would be otherwise suitable to add to a carbohydrate meal, the sugar content

on the nutritional label should be less than 4 grams per 100 gram serving.

2. For products that would be otherwise suitable to add to a protein meal, the sugar content on the nutritional label should be less than 1 gram per 100 gram serving.

T   **Thickeners**

Thickeners such as arrowroot and cornflour are highly refined from dense carbohydrates. They may cause the food you have thickened to have a high GI. For this reason we advise that you avoid using thickeners when cooking. Tricks for thickening food include condensing fluids by cooking with the lid off, or adding okra (a small green vegetable available from specialty fruit and vegetable stores) which has a natural thickening effect.

Tomato passata

The brands I use are Annalisa and LaGina. Both come from Italy and it's the way the Italians process the tomatos that gives them a low GI. So look for the Italian brands and make sure they have no added sugar. Read the section on sugar for more information on choosing brands.

	Tomato paste	There are brands that are sugar-free. Currently I am using Leggos, however you should always check the label. Read the section on sugar for more information on choosing brands.
V	Vinegar	Please don't use balsamic vinegar as it has caramel added to it that can cause your weight loss to plateau. Use other vinegars in moderation such as white wine vinegar, red wine vinegar and plain white vinegar.

Day 0 Shopping and cooking

Shopping

Vegetables	Fruit	
4 white onions	2 serves of fruit	1 tblsp white wine vinegar
3½ brown onions	1 lemon	300ml (1¼ cups) olive oil
16 spring onions	**Meat and seafood**	1 tblsp peanut oil
9½ sticks of celery	500g (16oz) lean beef mince	1 tsp sesame oil
4 garlic cloves		1 tblsp baby capers
2 medium eggplants	850g (28oz) chicken mince	415g (14½ oz) canned salmon
300g (9½oz) Swiss brown mushrooms	4 bacon rashers	400g (14oz) canned diced tomatoes
8 button mushrooms	300g (9½oz) diced lamb	1 cup tomato passata
2 Lebanese cucumbers		2 tblsp tomato paste
1 cucumber	**Dairy case**	12 eggs
200g (7oz) green beans	200g (7oz) grated tasty cheese	2 serves of nuts
6 tomatoes	½ cup grated Parmesan cheese	7 cups rolled oats
20 cherry tomatoes		2½ cups all-bran
2 cups wom bok	4 tblsp mascarpone	¼ cup unprocessed oat-bran
300g (9½oz) baby spinach leaves	1 tblsp butter	½ cup coarse oatmeal
2 cups rocket leaves	4 serves of cheese	1 cup dried apricots
1 small red chilli		1 litre malt-free soymilk
10 basil leaves	**Grocery**	Tea, decaffeinated coffee or herbal tea
8 rosemary stems	6 bay leaves	
½ cup dill	½ tsp dried oregano	
¼ cup tarragon	Sea salt	
3 cups flat-leaf parsley	Black pepper	
	1 tsp ground allspice	
	2 tsp ground cumin	
	½ tsp sambal oelek	
	½ tsp cinnamon	
	20 black peppercorns	
	1 tblsp red wine vinegar	

NB: For quantities and types of fruit, nuts and cheese, refer to the explanation in the recipe section of this book. For the best tea, decaffeinated coffee or herbal tea, see beverages in the recipe section.

Cooking

Vegetable stock: Make 2 lots of this recipe and freeze in 2 separate microwave-proof containers. To reheat frozen stock, place in the microwave for 9 minutes on high, stir twice during heating.

Apricot muesli: This muesli recipe will make enough for 2 people for 4–5 breakfasts each. On the meal planner it should last about 1½ weeks. Keep your muesli in an airtight container and serve it preferably with soymilk. You can top your muesli with fruit such as apricot or pear pieces in natural juice; this would add to your fruit tally.

Moussaka: This recipe makes enough for 2 people for 3 servings each. Once cooked, allow moussaka to cool slightly then cut into four pieces and place into individual freezer- and microwave-proof containers. Freeze until ready to use. For reheating defrosted servings of moussaka, place in the microwave for 6 minutes on high.

Salmon muffins: This recipe makes enough salmon muffins for 2 people for 1 dinner and 1 snack each. Once cooked, allow the salmon muffins to cool slightly before placing into a container for freezing. Freeze until ready to use. To reheat when defrosted, place in the microwave for 2 minutes on high. To reheat when frozen, place in the microwave for 6 minutes on high.

Chicken burgers: This recipe makes enough chicken burgers for 2 people for 2 lunches each. Once cooked, allow the chicken burgers to cool slightly before placing into a container for freezing. Freeze until ready to use. To reheat defrosted 4 piece servings of chicken burgers, place in the microwave for 3 minutes on high.

Tomato sauce with oregano: This recipe makes enough sauce to serve with 2 snacks each for 2 people. Keep it refrigerated until ready for use.

Day 1 Monday

Menu

Meal	Type	Meal solution
Breakfast	Protein	Swiss brown mushrooms served on wilted baby English spinach leaves
Lunch	Protein	Moussaka served with a salad with feta, cherry tomatoes and cucumber
Snack	Protein	Fresh vegetable snack served with tomato sauce with oregano
Dinner	Protein	Salmon muffins served with tomato and basil salad

Instructions

Time	What to do
Breakfast	• Cook *Swiss brown mushrooms served on wilted baby English spinach leaves* • Prepare *Salad with feta, cherry tomatoes and cucumber* and pack to take to work • Pack *Moussaka* to take to work • Pack *Fresh vegetable snack* and *Tomato sauce with oregano* to take to work • Refrigerate food once at work
Lunch	• Reheat the defrosted *Moussaka* for 6 minutes in the microwave on high, serve with the *Salad with feta, cherry tomatoes and cucumber*
Dinner	• Prepare the *Tomato and basil salad* • Reheat the frozen *Salmon muffins* (5 each) for 6 minutes in the microwave on high

Day 2 Tuesday

Menu

Meal	Type	Meal solution
Breakfast	Protein	*Bacon and eggs*
Lunch	Protein	*Chicken burgers served with cucumber and caper salad*
Snack	Protein	*Fresh vegetable snack served with tomato sauce with oregano and a serve of cheese*
Dinner	Protein	*Lamb stir-fry*

Instructions

Time	What to do
Breakfast	• Cook *Bacon and eggs* • Prepare *Cucumber and caper salad* and pack to take to work • Pack *Chicken burgers* (4 each) to take to work • Pack *Fresh vegetable snack* and *Tomato sauce with oregano* and *Cheese* to take to work • Refrigerate food once at work
Lunch	• Reheat the defrosted *Chicken burgers* (4 each) for 3 minutes in the microwave on high, serve with the *Cucumber and caper salad*
Dinner	• Prepare the *Lamb stir-fry* and serve

Day 3 Wednesday

Menu

Meal	Type	Meal solution
Breakfast	Carbohydrate	Apricot muesli with a serve of fruit

Wait at least three hours after breakfast before eating lunch

Meal	Type	Meal solution
Lunch	Protein	Moussaka with simple rocket salad
Snack	Protein	Serve of cheese and a serve of nuts
Dinner	Protein	Spicy chicken stir-fry

Instructions

Time	What to do
Breakfast	• Prepare *Simple rocket salad* and pack to take to work • Pack *Moussaka* to take to work • Pack *Cheese* and *Nuts* to take to work • Refrigerate food once at work
Lunch	• Reheat the defrosted *Moussaka* for 6 minutes in the microwave on high, serve with the *Simple rocket salad*
Dinner	• Prepare the *Spicy chicken stir-fry* and serve

Day 3 Shopping and cooking

Shopping

Vegetables	Fruit	Grocery
2 red onions	6 serves of fruit	4 tblsp mixed dried
1 brown onion	1 lemon	herbs
6 small shallots	1 lime	1½ tsp dried
1 spring onion		oregano
2½ garlic cloves	**Meat and seafood**	¼ tsp chilli powder
2 long red chillies	4 slices of	Sea salt
2¼ red capsicums	prosciutto	Black pepper
1 stick celery	750g (24oz) boned	150ml (5fl oz) white
14 Roma tomatoes	pork loin roll	wine vinegar
10 cherry tomatoes		2 tblsp red wine
2 baby fennel	**Dairy case**	vinegar
2 Lebanese	¼ cup butter	250ml (1 cup) olive
eggplants	2 serves of cheese	oil
6 asparagus spears	400g (14oz) hard	3 tsp baby capers
1 zucchini	tofu	1½ tsp tamarind
4 baby yellow	150g (5oz) haloumi	puree
squash	cheese	3 cups tomato
½ cucumber	50g (1½oz) feta	passata
¼ continental	cheese	800g (28oz) canned
cucumber	300g (9½oz) fresh	diced tomato
16 button	pasta	6 canned artichoke
mushrooms	1 tblsp sour cream	hearts
2 cups rocket		1¼ cups basmati
2 cups mixed		rice
lettuce		350g (12oz) white
¼ cup Thai basil		beans
4 tblsp Vietnamese		2 tblsp walnut
mint		pieces
¼ cup basil		5 eggs
½ cup coriander		20 slices of bread
1 cup flat-leaf		2 litres (8 cups)
parsley		malt-free soymilk

NB: For quantities and types of fruit, nuts and cheese servings, refer to the explanation in the recipe section of this book. For selecting the correct bread, refer to the explanation in the recipe section of this book.

Cooking

Basmati rice salad with tomatoes, fennel and fresh herbs:
Makes enough for 2 people for 2 meals each. Keep refrigerated.

Baked beans: Double the ingredients in this recipe to make enough for 2 people for 5 serves each. Freeze in 5 double-serve lots in microwave- and freezer-proof containers. For reheating when frozen, place in the microwave for 6 minutes on high, stir once during heating.

Tofu balls with tamarind and tomato sauce: Makes 32 tofu balls to have 5 per person for 2 lunches and 3 per person for 2 snacks. Tofu balls should be frozen with plastic separating them so you can easily remove the quantity you require to defrost for lunches and snacks. The tamarind and tomato sauce can be kept in the refrigerator in a sealed container. Serve cold or hot. For reheating tofu balls, place in the microwave for 2 minutes on high. For reheating the tamarind and tomato sauce, place the required amount of sauce in the microwave for 20–30 seconds.

Day 4 Thursday

Menu

Meal	Type	Meal solution
Breakfast	Carbohydrate	Apricot muesli
Lunch	Carbohydrate	Basmati rice salad with tomatoes, fennel and fresh herbs
Snack	Carbohydrate	One serve of fruit

Wait at least three hours after your snack before eating dinner

Meal	Type	Meal solution
Dinner	Protein	Barbecued haloumi and vegetables with lemon and capers

Instructions

Time	What to do
Breakfast	• Pack *Basmati rice salad with tomatoes, fennel and fresh herbs* and a serve of *Fruit* to take to work • Refrigerate food once at work
Dinner	• Prepare the *Barbecued haloumi and vegetables with lemon and capers* and serve

Day 5 Friday

Menu

Meal	Type	Meal solution
Breakfast	Carbohydrate	Baked beans on toast

Wait at least three hours after breakfast before eating lunch

Meal	Type	Meal solution
Lunch	Protein	Chicken burgers served with salad of rocket, walnuts and feta
Snack	Protein	Salmon muffins
Dinner	Protein	Vegetable kebabs served with tomato salsa

Instructions

Time	What to do
Breakfast	• Reheat *Baked beans* and cook *Performax toast* for breakfast • Prepare *Salad of rocket, walnuts and feta* and pack for work • Pack *Chicken burgers* (4 each) for work • Pack *Salmon muffins* for work • Refrigerate food at work
Lunch	• Reheat the defrosted *Chicken burgers* (4 each) for 3 minutes in the microwave on high, serve with the *Salad of rocket, walnuts and feta*
Snack	• Reheat the defrosted *Salmon Muffins* for 2 minutes in the microwave on high
Dinner	• Prepare *Vegetable kebabs* and *Tomato salsa* and serve

Day 6 Saturday

Menu

Meal	Type	Meal solution
Breakfast	Carbohydrate	Apricot muesli
Lunch	Carbohydrate	Tofu balls with tamarind and tomato sauce served with an Asian salad
Snack	Carbohydrate	One serve of fruit

Wait at least three hours after your snack before eating dinner

Meal	Type	Meal solution
Dinner	Protein	Fresh pasta with passata, capers and parsley

Instructions

Time	What to do
Breakfast	• Remove required *Tofu balls* (5 each) from the freezer and place in the refrigerator to defrost
Lunch	• Prepare *Asian salad* and serve with the *Tofu balls with tamarind and tomato sauce*. If desired you can serve the *Tofu balls* heated; heat the defrosted *Tofu balls* in the microwave for 2 minutes on high. Heat the required amount of sauce for 20–30 seconds in the microwave on high
Dinner	• Prepare *Fresh pasta with passata, capers and parsley* and serve

Day 7 Sunday

Menu

Meal	Type	Meal solution
Breakfast	Protein	Grilled haloumi, Roma tomatoes and prosciutto served with scrambled eggs

Wait at least five hours after breakfast before eating lunch

Meal	Type	Meal solution
Lunch	Carbohydrate	Basmati rice salad with tomatoes, fennel and fresh herbs served with a piece of fruit

Wait at least three hours after lunch before eating your snack

Meal	Type	Meal solution
Snack	Protein	Fresh vegetable snack and a serve of cheese
Dinner	Protein	Roast pork served with roasted red onion and Roma tomatoes and Hollandaise sauce

Instructions

Time	What to do
Breakfast	• Cook *Grilled haloumi, Roma tomatoes and prosciutto served with scrambled eggs*
Dinner	• Cook *Roast pork* and *Roasted red onion and Roma tomatoes* and *Hollandaise sauce* and serve

Day 7 Shopping and cooking

Shopping

Vegetables		Grocery
1¼ red onions	¼ cup coriander	Sea salt
½ brown onion	¼ cup Thai basil	Black pepper
3 garlic cloves	2 tblsp Vietnamese	220ml (7½fl oz)
1 tsp grated ginger	mint	olive oil
¾ long red chilli		2 tblsp white wine
¼ red capsicum	**Fruit**	vinegar
300g (9½oz) Swiss	4 serves of fruit	16 eggs
brown mushrooms	2 lemons	415g (14½oz)
10 button	1 lime	canned salmon
mushrooms		2 serves of nuts
8 sun-dried	**Meat and seafood**	1 litre (4 cups)
tomatoes	2 rindless bacon	malt-free soymilk
18 cherry tomatoes	rashers	Tea, decaffeinated
1 tomato	2 large white fish	coffee or herbal
4 Roma tomatoes	fillets	tea
100g (3½oz) green	2 chicken breast	
beans	fillets	
1½ sticks of celery		
½ Lebanese	**Dairy case**	
cucumber	1 cup grated cheese	
½ cucumber	¼ cup grated	
¼ continental	Parmesan cheese	
cucumber	4 tblsp mascarpone	
500g (16oz) baby	50g (1½oz) feta	
spinach leaves	cheese	
4 cups mixed salad	4 serves of cheese	
leaves	1 tblsp butter	
2 cups rocket		
¾ cup flat-leaf		
parsley		
½ cup dill		
¼ cup tarragon		
10 basil leaves		

NB: For quantities and types of fruit, nuts and cheese, refer to the explanation in the recipe section of this book. For the best tea, decaffeinated coffee or herbal tea, see beverages in the recipe section.

Cooking

Frittata with bacon and sun-dried tomatoes: This recipe makes enough for 2 people for 2 serves each. Freeze in microwave- and freezer-proof containers in 4 single serve portions. For re-heating when defrosted, place in the microwave for 6 minutes on high.

Salmon muffins: This recipe makes enough salmon muffins for 2 people for 1 dinner and 1 snack each. Once cooked, allow the salmon muffins to cool slightly before placing into a container for freezing. Freeze until ready to use. To reheat when defrosted, place in the microwave for 2 minutes on high. To reheat when frozen, place in the microwave for 6 minutes on high.

Day 8 Monday

Menu

Meal	Type	Meal solution
Breakfast	Carbohydrate	Apricot muesli with a serve of fruit

**Wait at least three hours after breakfast
before eating lunch**

Meal	Type	Meal solution
Lunch	Protein	Moussaka served with salad with feta, cherry tomatoes and cucumber
Snack	Protein	Fresh vegetable snack and serve of cheese
Dinner	Protein	Salmon muffins served with simple rocket salad

Instructions

Time	What to do
Breakfast	• Prepare *Salad with feta, cherry tomatoes and cucumber* and pack for work • Pack *Moussaka* for work • Pack *Fresh vegetable snack* and *Cheese* for work • Refrigerate food at work
Lunch	• Reheat defrosted *Moussaka* 6 minutes in the microwave on high, serve with the *Salad with feta, cherry tomatoes and cucumber*
Dinner	• Prepare *Simple rocket salad* • Reheat the frozen *Salmon muffins* (5 each) for 6 minutes in the microwave on high, serve with the *Simple rocket salad*

Day 9 Tuesday

Menu

Meal	Type	Meal solution
Breakfast	Carbohydrate	*Baked beans on toast*

Wait at least three hours after breakfast before eating lunch

Meal	Type	Meal solution
Lunch	Protein	*Frittata with bacon and sun-dried tomatoes served with tomato and basil salad*
Snack	Protein	*Serve of cheese and a serve of nuts*
Dinner	Protein	*Barbecued fish fillets served with tomato salsa*

Instructions

Time	What to do
Breakfast	• Reheat the frozen *Baked beans* in the microwave for 6 minutes on high, stir once during heating. Cook *Performax toast* and serve with the beans • Prepare *Tomato and basil salad* and pack for work • Pack *Frittata with bacon and sun-dried tomatoes* for work • Pack serve of *Cheese* and *Nuts* for work • Refrigerate food at work
Lunch	• Reheat the defrosted *Frittata with bacon and sun-dried tomatoes* 6 minutes in the microwave on high, serve with the *Tomato and basil salad*
Dinner	• Prepare *Tomato salsa* • Prepare *Barbecued fish fillets* and serve with the *Tomato salsa*

Day 10 Wednesday

Menu

Meal	Type	Meal solution
Breakfast	Protein	Swiss brown mushrooms served on wilted baby English spinach

Wait at least five hours after breakfast before eating lunch

Meal	Type	Meal solution
Lunch	Carbohydrate	Tofu balls with tamarind and tomato sauce served with an Asian salad
Snack	Carbohydrate	One serve of fruit

Wait at least three hours after your snack before eating dinner

Meal	Type	Meal solution
Dinner	Protein	Chicken soup

Instructions

Time	What to do
Breakfast	• Prepare *Swiss brown mushrooms served on wilted baby English spinach* and serve • Pack *Tofu balls* (5 each) *with tamarind and tomato sauce* for work • Prepare *Asian salad* and pack for work • Pack a serve of *Fruit* for work
Lunch	• If desired, the *Tofu balls with tomato and tamarind sauce* can be served heated. Heat the *Tofu balls* in the microwave for 2 minutes on high. Heat the required amount of *Tomato and tamarind sauce* in the microwave for 20–30 seconds.
Dinner	• Prepare *Chicken soup* and serve

Day 10 Shopping and cooking

Shopping

Vegetables	Fruit	Grocery
3 browns onions	6 serves of fruit	Sea salt
1½ red onions	1 lemon	Black pepper
5½ garlic cloves	½ lime	1 tsp turmeric
2½ long red chillies		½ tsp paprika
2 tomatoes	**Meat and seafood**	1 tsp ground
4 Roma tomatoes	250g (8oz) mince	coriander
6 button mushrooms	beef	¼ tsp chilli powder
2 sticks of celery	6 lamb cutlets	1 tsp Cajun seasoning
100g (3½oz) green	4 bacon rashers	2 tsp cumin
beans	450g (15½oz) lean	1½ tblsp dried
4 Lebanese eggplants	beef strips	oregano
1 red capsicum		1 cup tomato passata
1 head of broccoli	**Dairy case**	800g (28oz) canned
4 zucchini	2 serves of cheese	diced tomatoes
6 baby yellow squash	100g (3½ oz) feta	400g (14oz) canned
4 asparagus spears	cheese	red kidney beans
2 sweet potatoes	300g (9½oz) fresh	2 canned artichoke
½ cucumber	pasta	hearts
2 cups rocket		2 tsp baby capers
2 tblsps basil		420ml (1¾ cups)
¾ cup coriander		olive oil
¾ cup parsley		2 tblsp red wine
		vinegar
		2 tblsp walnut pieces
		5 eggs
		1 cup dried apricots
		7 cups rolled oats
		2½ cups all-bran
		¼ cup unprocessed
		oat-bran
		¼ cup unprocessed
		barley bran
		½ cup coarse oat
		meal
		2 litres (8 cups) malt-
		free soymilk

NB: For quantities and types of fruit, nuts and cheese servings, refer to the explanation in the recipe section of this book.

Cooking

Apricot muesli: This muesli recipe will make enough for 2 people for 4-5 breakfasts each. On the meal planner it should last about 1½ weeks. Keep your muesli in an airtight container and serve it preferably with soy milk. You can top your muesli with fruit such as apricot or pear pieces in natural juice; this would add to your fruit tally.

Spicy vegetable soup with red kidney beans and coriander: This recipe makes enough for 2 people for 3 serves each. Keep frozen in microwave- and freezer-proof containers in 6 individual serves. To reheat when defrosted, place in the microwave for 5 minutes on high.

Day 11 Thursday

Menu

Meal	Type	Meal solution
Breakfast	Carbohydrate	*Apricot muesli and a serve of fruit*
Lunch	Carbohydrate	*Spicy vegetable soup with red kidney beans and coriander*

Wait at least three hours after lunch before eating your snack

Meal	Type	Meal solution
Snack	Protein	*Serve of cheese*
Dinner	Protein	*Middle Eastern burgers served with a Greek salad*

Instructions

Time	What to do
Breakfast	• Pack *Spicy vegetable soup with red kidney beans and coriander* for work • Pack a serve of *Cheese* for work • Refrigerate food at work
Lunch	• Reheat defrosted *Spicy vegetable soup with red kidney beans and coriander* soup 5 minutes in the microwave on high and serve
Dinner	• Prepare *Greek salad* • Cook *Middle Eastern burgers* and serve with the *Greek salad*

Day 12 Friday

Menu

Meal	Type	Meal solution
Breakfast	Carbohydrate	Apricot muesli and a serve of fruit

Wait at least three hours after breakfast before eating lunch

Meal	Type	Meal solution
Lunch	Protein	Frittata with bacon and sun-dried tomatoes served with salad of rocket, walnuts and feta
Snack	Protein	Salmon muffins
Dinner	Protein	Vegetable salad served with tomato salsa

Instructions

Time	What to do
Breakfast	• Pack *Frittata with bacon and sun-dried tomatoes* for work • Prepare *Salad of rocket, walnuts and feta* and pack for work • Pack *Salmon muffins* for work • Refrigerate food at work
Lunch	• Reheat *Frittata with bacon and sun-dried tomatoes* for 6 minutes in the microwave on high, and serve with the *Salad of rocket, walnuts and feta*
Snack	• Reheat the defrosted *Salmon muffins* in the microwave for 2 minutes on high
Dinner	• Prepare *Vegetable salad* • Prepare *Tomato salsa* and serve with the *Vegetable salad*

Day 13 Saturday

Menu

Meal	Type	Meal solution
Breakfast	Carbohydrate	*Baked beans on toast*
Lunch	Carbohydrate	*Fresh pasta with passata, capers and parsley*
Snack	Carbohydrate	*Tofu balls with tamarind and tomato sauce*

Wait at least three hours after your snack before eating dinner

Meal	Type	Meal solution
Dinner	Protein	*Barbecued lamb cutlets served with barbecued vegetables*

Instructions

Time	What to do
Breakfast	• Reheat the frozen *Baked beans* in the microwave for 6 minutes on high, stir once during heating. Cook *Performax toast* and serve with the beans • Remove *Tofu balls* from the freezer and allow to defrost in the refrigerator for your afternoon snack
Lunch	• Prepare *Fresh pasta with passata, capers and parsley* and serve
Snack	• If desired the *Tofu balls with tomato and tamarind sauce* can be served heated. Heat the defrosted *Tofu balls* in the microwave for 2 minutes on high. Heat the required

amount of *Tomato and tamarind sauce* in the microwave for 20–30 seconds

Dinner
• Cook *Barbecued lamb cutlets* and *Barbecued vegetables* and serve

Day 14 Sunday

Menu

Meal	Type	Meal solution
Breakfast	Protein	*Bacon and eggs*

Wait at least five hours after breakfast before eating lunch

Meal	Type	Meal solution
Lunch	Carbohydrate	*Spicy vegetable soup with red kidney beans and coriander*
Snack	Carbohydrate	*One serve of fruit*

Wait at least three hours after your snack before eating dinner

Meal	Type	Meal solution
Dinner	Protein	*Cajun beef stir-fry*

Instructions

Time	What to do
Breakfast	• Cook *Bacon and eggs* and serve • Place two servings of the *Spicy vegetable soup with red kidney beans and coriander* in the refrigerator to defrost
Lunch	• Re-heat each serving of the defrosted *Spicy vegetable soup with red kidney beans and coriander* in the microwave for 5 minutes on high and serve
Dinner	• Cook *Cajun beef stir-fry* and serve

Day 14 Shopping and cooking

Shopping

Vegetables	Fruit	Grocery
1 red onion	6 serves of fruit	½ tsp cinnamon
4 spring onions	1 lemon	Sea salt
4 garlic cloves		Black pepper
2 tsp grated ginger	**Meat and seafood**	1 tblsp mixed herbs
8 oyster mushrooms	1 squid hood	420ml (1¾ cup)
400g (14oz) Swiss	2 baby octopus	olive oil
brown mushrooms	100g (3½oz) prawn	2 cups basmati rice
8 button mush-	meat	190g (6½oz) canned
rooms	1 white fish fillet	whole
20 cherry tomatoes	2 chicken breasts	champignons
10 sun-dried		1½ tblsp baby
tomatoes	**Dairy case**	capers
1 stick of celery	500g (16oz) ricotta	2 tblsp walnut
1 red capsicum	¾ cup mozzarella	pieces
2 Lebanese eggplants	¼ cup Parmesan	20g (½oz) pecans
6 asparagus spears	cheese	2 eggs
1 zucchini	100g (3½oz) feta	250g (8oz) frozen
2 baby yellow squash	cheese	spinach
½ cucumber	100g (3½oz) haloumi	2 litres (8 cups)
2½ Lebanese	2 serves cheese	malt-free soymilk
cucumbers	1 tblsp butter	Tea, decaffeinated
250g (8oz) baby		coffee or herbal
English spinach		tea
2 cups rocket		
4 cups mixed salad		
leaves		
½ cup parsley		
1 tblsp mint		
¾ cup coriander		

NB: For quantities and types of fruit, nuts and cheese, refer to the explanation in the recipe section of this book. For the best tea, decaffeinated coffee or herbal tea, see beverages in the recipe section.

Cooking

Spinach and ricotta tarts: This recipe makes enough for 2 people for 2 meals each. The recipe makes 16 tarts in total, 4 for each meal. Freeze the tarts in a freezer-proof container with plastic wrap between them for ease of separation. Serve hot or cold. To reheat serves of 4 defrosted tarts, place in the microwave for 2 minutes on high.

Mushroom risotto: This recipe makes enough for 2 people for 2 meals each. Divide into 4 freezer-proof containers and freeze. To reheat defrosted individual servings, place in the microwave for 3 minutes on high, stir once during heating.

Day 15 Monday

Menu

Meal	Type	Meal solution
Breakfast	Carbohydrate	Apricot muesli and a serve of fruit

Wait at least three hours after breakfast before eating lunch

Meal	Type	Meal solution
Lunch	Protein	Spinach and ricotta tarts served with cucumber and caper salad
Snack	Protein	Fresh vegetable snack and a serve of cheese
Dinner	Protein	Stir-fried seafood served with salad of rocket, walnuts and feta

Instructions

Time	What to do
Breakfast	• Prepare *Caper and cucumber salad* and pack for work • Pack *Spinach and ricotta tarts* (4 each) for work • Pack *Fresh vegetable snack* and *Cheese* for work • Refrigerate food at work
Lunch	• To reheat defrosted serves of *Spinach and ricotta tarts* (4 each), place in the microwave for 2 minutes on high, serve with *Cucumber and caper salad*
Dinner	• Prepare *Salad of rocket, walnuts and feta* • Cook *Stir-fried seafood* and serve with the *Salad of rocket, walnuts and feta*

Day 16 Tuesday

Menu

Meal	Type	Meal solution
Breakfast	Protein	*Swiss brown mushrooms served on wilted baby English spinach leaves*

Wait at least five hours after breakfast before eating lunch

Meal	Type	Meal solution
Lunch	Carbohydrate	*Mushroom risotto*
Snack	Carbohydrate	*One serve of fruit*

Wait at least three hours after your snack before eating dinner

Meal	Type	Meal solution
Dinner	Protein	*Barbecued haloumi and vegetables with lemon and capers*

Instructions

Time	What to do
Breakfast	• Cook *Swiss brown mushrooms served on wilted baby English spinach leaves* and serve for breakfast • Pack *Mushroom risotto* for work • Pack one serve of *Fruit* for work • Refrigerate food at work
Lunch	• Reheat defrosted *Mushroom risotto* for 3 minutes in the microwave on high
Dinner	• Cook *Barbecued haloumi and vegetables with lemon and caper dressing* and serve

Day 17 Wednesday

Menu

Meal	Type	Meal solution
Breakfast	Carbohydrate	Apricot muesli and a serve of fruit
Lunch	Carbohydrate	Spicy vegetable soup with red kidney beans and coriander
Snack	Carbohydrate	Tofu balls with tomato and tamarind sauce

Wait at least three hours after your snack before eating dinner

Meal	Type	Meal solution
Dinner	Protein	Chicken and pecan salad with lemon aioli

Instructions

Time	What to do
Breakfast	• Pack *Spicy vegetable soup with red kidney beans and coriander* for work • Pack *Tofu balls* (3 each) *with tomato and tamarind sauce* for work • Refrigerate food at work
Lunch	• Reheat defrosted *Spicy vegetable soup with red kidney beans and coriander* for 5 minutes on high in the microwave, then serve
Snack	• If desired the *Tofu balls with tomato and tamarind sauce* can be served heated. Heat the defrosted *Tofu balls* in the microwave for 2 minutes on high. Heat the required

amount of *Tomato and tamarind sauce* in
the microwave for 20–30 seconds

Dinner   • Cook *Chicken and pecan salad with lemon
aioli* and serve

Day 17 Shopping and cooking

Shopping

Vegetables	Fruit	Grocery
½ red onion	4 serves of fruit	1½ tsp dried
2 spring onions	2½ lemons	oregano
4 garlic cloves		1 star anise
1 slice of ginger	**Meat and seafood**	1 cinnamon stick
30 cherry tomatoes	2 beef round	2 cloves
1 tomato	medallions	Sea salt
3 Roma tomatoes	8 slices of prosciutto	Black pepper
8 sun-dried	700g (23oz)	350ml (1½ cups)
tomatoes	boneless lamb leg	olive oil
12 button	roast, in a roll	1 tblsp peanut oil
mushrooms	400g (14oz) diced	1 tsp sesame oil
6 asparagus spears	pork	5 tblsp red wine
1 baby yellow squash		vinegar
1 zucchini	**Dairy case**	1 tblsp white wine
3 cups wom bok	6 servings of cheese	vinegar
2 cups bean shoots	300g (9½oz) fresh	2 cups tomato
2 sticks of celery	pasta	passata
1 cucumber	110g (3½oz) feta	1½ tsp baby capers
1½ Lebanese	cheese	3 canned anchovies
cucumbers	50g (1½oz) haloumi	200g (7oz) canned
4 cups rocket	cheese	sardines in oil
5 cups mixed salad	1 tblsp sour cream	10 eggs
1 cup parsley	¼ cup butter	2 litres(8 cups) malt
8 basil leaves		free soymilk
4 tblsps thyme		

NB: For quantities and types of fruit, nuts and cheese servings, refer to the explanation in the recipe section of this book.

Cooking

Tomato sauce with oregano: This recipe makes enough sauce to serve with 2 snacks each for 2 people. Keep it refrigerated until ready for use.

Day 18 Thursday

Menu

Meal	Type	Meal solution
Breakfast	Carbohydrate	*Baked beans on toast*

Wait at least three hours after breakfast before eating lunch

Meal	Type	Meal solution
Lunch	Protein	*Spinach and ricotta tarts served with a simple rocket salad*
Snack	Protein	*Fresh vegetable snack served with tomato sauce with oregano and a serve of cheese*
Dinner	Protein	*Beef round medallions served with salsa verde salad*

Instructions

Time	What to do
Breakfast	• Reheat the frozen *Baked beans* in the microwave for 6 minutes on high, stir once during heating. Cook *Performax toast* and serve with the beans • Pack *Spinach and ricotta tarts* (4 each) for work • Prepare and pack *Simple rocket salad* for work • Pack *Fresh vegetable snack* and *Tomato sauce with oregano* and a serve of *Cheese* for work • Refrigerate food at work

Lunch	• To reheat defrosted serves of *Spinach and ricotta tarts* (4 each), place in the microwave for 2 minutes on high, serve with the *Simple rocket salad*
Dinner	• Prepare *Salsa verde salad* • Cook *Beef round medallions* and serve with the *Salsa verde salad* for dinner

Day 19 Friday

Menu

Meal	Type	Meal solution
Breakfast	Carbohydrate	Apricot muesli with one serve of fruit
Lunch	Carbohydrate	Mushroom risotto
Snack	Carbohydrate	One serve of fruit
Dinner	Carbohydrate	Fresh pasta with passata, capers and parsley

Instructions

Time	What to do
Breakfast	• Pack *Mushroom risotto* for work • Pack a serve of *Fruit* for work • Refrigerate food at work
Lunch	• Reheat *Mushroom risotto* for 3 minutes in the microwave on high
Dinner	• Cook *Fresh pasta with passata, capers and parsley* and serve

Day 20 Saturday

Menu

Meal	Type	Meal solution
Breakfast	Carbohydrate	Baked beans on toast

Wait at least three hours after breakfast before eating lunch

Meal	Type	Meal solution
Lunch	Protein	Egg roll-ups
Snack	Protein	Fresh vegetable snack served with tomato sauce with oregano and a serve of cheese
Dinner	Protein	Roast lamb served with roast vegetables and Hollandaise sauce

Instructions

Time	What to do
Breakfast	• Reheat the frozen *Baked beans* in the microwave for 6 minutes on high, stir once during heating. Cook *Performax toast* and serve with the beans
Lunch	• Cook *Egg roll-ups* and serve
Dinner	• Cook *Roast lamb* and *Roast vegetables* and *Hollandaise sauce* and serve

Day 21 Sunday

Menu

Meal	Type	Meal solution
Breakfast	Protein	*Grilled haloumi, Roma tomatoes and prosciutto served with scrambled eggs*
Lunch	Protein	*Salad with sardine fillets*
Snack	Protein	*Serve of cheese*
Dinner	Protein	*Asian pork stir-fry*

Instructions

Time	What to do
Breakfast	• Cook *Grilled haloumi, Roma tomatoes and prosciutto served with scrambled eggs* and serve
Lunch	• Cook *Salad with sardine fillets* and serve
Dinner	• Cook *Asian pork stir-fry* and serve

Finishing the meal planner

Now that you have finished the 21-day meal planner and have completed all your health goals for this three-week period, congratulate yourself on your achievement. You are experienced at cooking all the recipes, so you can do the three weeks over again. There is nothing stopping you, there is plenty of variety and you'll be a wiz at it.

My suggestion is that you incorporate this style of eating into your regular diet to maintain your health throughout your entire life. There are many more recipes available in our cookbooks, and through our website at www.glycemic-index.com, to enable your tastebuds to be well looked after for some time to come. By maintaining this healthy lifestyle you may dramatically increase your chances of avoiding such problems as diabetes, heart disease, high cholesterol and cancer, not to mention increasing your longevity and maintaining a youthful appearance.

Recipes

Stocks and sauces
Breakfast, beverages and breads
Snacks and side-dishes
Mains

STOCKS AND SAUCES

Vegetable stock

Tomato sauce with oregano

Hollandaise sauce

Vegetable stock
Carbohydrate/Protein

Use this stock for the soup and risotto recipes in this book. It is easy to make and you can keep it frozen for later use if required.

When following the meal planner you will need to make 2 lots of this recipe and freeze in 2 separate microwave-proof containers. To reheat frozen stock, place in the microwave for 9 minutes on high, stir twice during heating.

2 white onions and skins, finely chopped
8 whole spring onions, finely chopped
1 cup parsley and stalks, chopped
4 stems of rosemary
3 sticks celery and leaves, chopped
3 bay leaves
10 black peppercorns
½ small red chilli, seeded and chopped (optional)
Any of the following if available, chopped roughly (save
    your kitchen scraps): broccoli stems, cabbage outer
    leaves, cauliflower stems and leaves, leftover zucchini
2.5 litres (10 cups) of water
Sea salt to taste

Place all ingredients, except the salt, in a large saucepan. Cover, then bring to the boil; reduce heat and simmer gently for 1½ hours. Strain off liquid and discard solids. Lightly season with salt. Keep refrigerated.

Total cooking time: 15 minutes preparation, 1½ hours cooking
Makes: 1¾ (7 cups) litres of stock

Tomato sauce with oregano

Carbohydrate/Protein

You can serve this sauce with either protein- or carbohydrate-style meals. It is excellent served as a dipping sauce with the 'fresh vegetable snacks' in the snacks and side-dishes section.

When following the meal planner this recipe makes enough sauce to serve with 2 snacks each for 2 people. Keep it refrigerated until ready for use.

1 cup tomato passata
½ teaspoon dried oregano
1 tablespoon red wine vinegar
Sea salt and freshly cracked black pepper to taste

Combine all ingredients in a small saucepan; bring to the boil then reduce heat and allow to simmer for 5 minutes or until sauce has thickened.

Total cooking time: 10 minutes
Makes: ½ cup sauce

Hollandaise sauce

Protein

This sauce is excellent for serving with roasts. The trick to this recipe is to heat it very slowly and to have lots of patience.

1 egg yolk
2 teaspoons water
¼ cup butter, melted
½ teaspoon lemon juice
Sea salt and freshly ground black pepper to taste

Whisk egg yolks and water together over a very low heat for
2 minutes or until thick and foamy. Remove from heat. Slowly pour
melted butter into the egg yolk mixture, whisking continually to form
a thick and creamy sauce. Stir through lemon juice and seasoning.
If sauce is runny, return to low heat and whisk until thickened.
Try pouring Hollandaise sauce over your next roast.

Total cooking time: 15 minutes preparation
Makes: 1 cup

BREAKFAST, BEVERAGES AND BREADS

Beverages

Sparkling orange and grapefruit juice with ginger

Tomato and celery juice with parsley

Apricot muesli

Grilled haloumi, Roma tomatoes and prosciutto served with scrambled eggs

Bacon and eggs

Baked beans on toast

Swiss brown mushrooms served on wilted baby English spinach leaves

Beverages

Fruit juice: Carbohydrate

Remember the same time window rules apply to beverages so drink your juice with your carbohydrate meals only. Juice is a moderate carbohydrate so remember that you should only have moderate carbohydrates in moderation. Only drink juice clearly labelled as having no added sugar, or make your own. Apple juice, orange juice and grapefruit juice are all acceptable. See an example of fruit juice in the following pages.

Vegetable juice: Carbohydrate or Carbohydrate/Protein

When juicing vegetables use only moderate and good carbohydrate vegetables. Moderate carbohydrate vegetables, such as sweet potato, will make juices that you should only drink with carbohydrate meals. Good carbohydrate vegetables such as tomato and celery will make juices that you can drink with either a carbohydrate or a protein meal. See examples of vegetable juice in the following pages.

Tea: Carbohydrate/Protein

Only use tea that is low caffeine. We use a brand called 'Madura' which is 3% caffeine. This is acceptable. Please note that green tea, like most black tea, does have caffeine. You can use a little soymilk in your tea but do not add sugar. See the section on artificial sweeteners if you are thinking about adding them to your tea.

Herbal tea: Carbohydrate/Protein

Most herbal teas are caffeine free and therefore suitable to have with any meal. Some suggested herbal teas include lemon, peppermint and camomile. Avoid the fruit flavoured and liquorice root teas as they may cause your weight to plateau. See the section on artificial sweeteners if you are thinking about adding them to your herbal tea.

Coffee: Carbohydrate/Protein

Use decaffeinated coffee only. You can use a little soy milk in your decaffeinated coffee but do not add any sugar. See the section on artificial sweeteners if you are thinking about adding them to your decaffeinated coffee.

Soymilk: Carbohydrate

Soymilk is the alternative to regular milk. Made from soy beans it is classified as a moderate carbohydrate, however adding small amounts to your tea and coffee is alright and shouldn't cause you any problems. Choose sugar-free soymilk that does not contain maltodextrine. Try to avoid drinking straight soymilk, being a moderate carbohydrate you should only use it in moderation. Some on your muesli in the morning and in your cups of tea should be fine.

Milk: Carbohydrate/Lipid

Milk is not allowed because it is a combination of sugar and fat together and from our experience guaranteed to hold up your progress. Excellent alternative sources of calcium are Parmesan cheese, canned salmon with bones and white beans, while spinach, broccoli, bok choy and soy beans also contribute to your recommended daily intake of calcium.

Beverages you should forget about are: cola drinks, soft drinks, milk drinks, goat's milk, sheep's milk, rice milk, cordial, sports drinks, flavoured yoghurt drinks, wine, beer, spirits, regular coffee and energy drinks.

Beverages you should become reacquainted with:

- WATER
- WATER
- WATER

Water is the most thirst-quenching substance known. You can drink water with any meal and at any time of the day. You should have at least 6–8 glasses of water per day. (N.B. Cups of tea and decaffeinated coffee will also count towards your water intake tally.)

Sparkling orange and grapefruit juice with ginger
Carbohydrate

2 grapefruit

2 oranges

½ teaspoon grated ginger

100ml (3½fl oz) sparkling mineral water

Juice the grapefruit and oranges and combine with the ginger and mineral water.

Total cooking time: 5 minutes preparation
Serves: 2

Tomato and celery juice with parsley

Carbohydrate/Protein

6 tomatoes

2 celery sticks

2 teaspoons lemon juice

2 tablespoons of fresh parsley

Juice all ingredients together in a juicer, or blend in a processor until smooth.

Total cooking time: 5 minutes preparation
Serves: 2

Apricot muesli
Carbohydrate

Oats are a good source of soluble and insoluble fibre. Insoluble fibre helps promote regular bowel motions whilst research suggests that the soluble fibre in oats contributes to lowering cholesterol. Use only rolled oats, not quick oats for this recipe. Quick oats have a greater surface area because they have been more finely ground – this increases the glycemic index.

I also use coarse oatmeal in this recipe to give it a more crunchy texture. You should be able to find the coarse oatmeal at your local health food store. If you are unable to get coarse oatmeal then just leave it out.

We recommend that you use malt-free soymilk on your muesli. You can top your muesli with fruit such as apricot or pear pieces in natural juice; this would add to your fruit tally. Read all about the fruit you can eat in the snacks and side-dishes section.

When following the meal planner this muesli recipe will make enough for 2 people for 4–5 breakfasts each. On the meal planner it should last about 1½ weeks. Keep your muesli in an airtight container.

7 cups rolled oats (not quick oats)
2½ cups all-bran
¼ cup unprocessed barley bran
¼ cup unprocessed oat bran
½ cup coarse oatmeal
1 cup dried apricots, diced

Combine all ingredients together and mix well. Store your muesli in a well-sealed container and it will keep for up to 2 weeks.

Total cooking time: 10 minutes preparation
Makes 10 bowls

Grilled haloumi, Roma tomatoes and prosciutto served with scrambled eggs

Protein

Haloumi cheese is a sheep's milk cheese traditionally made in Cyprus. It is quite salty so you may want to rinse it before grilling to wash away some of the salt. You can find this cheese in your supermarket or delicatessen.

2 Roma tomatoes, halved lengthways
50g (1.5oz) haloumi cheese, sliced 1cm thick
4 thin slices of prosciutto
4 tablespoons olive oil
½ teaspoon dried oregano
Sea salt and freshly cracked black pepper to taste

Scrambled eggs
4 eggs, lightly beaten
1 tablespoon sour cream
Sea salt and freshly cracked black pepper to taste
1 tablespoon olive oil
Fresh flat-leaf parsley to garnish

Toss together tomatoes, haloumi, prosciutto, olive oil, oregano and seasoning. Grill for 3–5 minutes under a hot grill; prosciutto should be crisp, tomatoes tender and haloumi browned on both sides.

For the scrambled eggs, combine eggs, sour cream and seasoning, whisk together well to combine. Heat oil in a small saucepan, add egg mixture and gently stir over medium heat until eggs are set.

Serve grilled tomatoes, haloumi and prosciutto with scrambled eggs to the side. Serve garnished with fresh flat-leaf parsley.

Total cooking time: 5 minutes preparation, 10 minutes cooking
Serves: 2

Bacon and eggs
Protein

1 tablespoon olive oil

4 eggs

4 rashers of bacon

Sea salt and freshly cracked black pepper to taste

Heat oil in a large frying pan. Crack eggs into the pan and cook over low heat for 5 minutes or until cooked as desired.

Grill bacon under a hot grill for 3–4 minutes each side or until cooked as desired.

Serve bacon and eggs onto warmed plates and season.

Total cooking time: 10 minutes cooking
Serves: 2

Baked beans on toast
Carbohydrate

For this recipe I use Great Northern beans otherwise known as 'white beans'. If you cannot find them then substitute with lima beans. Remember tomato passata is the pureed tomato in a jar, found near the tomato paste in the supermarket. White beans are a good source of calcium with 60 grams of cooked white beans yielding 30% of your recommended daily intake of calcium.

When selecting bread for your toast in this recipe, you should consult the explanation about bread in this recipe section and by referring to the index. I have suggested 2 types of bread that we have found to be suitable. Be cautious when choosing bread; remember 'when in doubt, leave it out.' Once you have found a suitable bread, you should keep it frozen until ready for use so it will last for the two-and-a-half weeks required.

When following the meal planner you should double the ingredients in this recipe to make enough for 2 people for 5 serves each. Freeze in 5 double-serve lots in microwave and freezer proof containers. For reheating when frozen, place in the microwave for 6 minutes on high, stir once during heating.

175g (6oz) dried white beans, soaked in cold water overnight, then drained

1 cup tomato passata

400g (14oz) diced tomatoes

½ onion, minced

1 tablespoon mixed dried herbs

2 tablespoons white wine vinegar

salt and freshly cracked pepper to taste

10 slices 'Performax' or 'Rye Hi-Soy and Linseed' bread
  by Country Life Bakery, or equivalent, either made
  from triticale or is low GI/low fat.

*Cook beans in a large saucepan of boiling water for 30 minutes; then
drain well. In a casserole dish combine beans, passata, tomatoes,
onion, herbs and vinegar. Cover casserole dish and cook at 180°C
(350°F) for 1 hour. Remove lid, season, then cook for a further
30 minutes or until the beans are soft and sauce has condensed.
Serve baked beans with slices of toasted Performax bread.*

*You can keep the baked beans in an airtight container in the
refrigerator for up to 5 days, or freeze in single servings. To reheat
frozen beans place in microwave on high for 6 minutes; stir twice
during cooking.*

Total cooking time: 12 hours soaking, 10 minutes preparation, 1½ hours cooking
Serves: 4

Swiss brown mushrooms served on wilted baby English spinach leaves

Protein

Swiss brown mushrooms have a stronger, more robust flavour than the normal white capped mushrooms. I use them in this recipe for this stronger flavour and to give variety for your tastebuds in the meal plan. If you are unable to find Swiss brown mushrooms then you can substitute with the normal white capped button mushrooms.

1 tablespoon butter
2 tablespoons olive oil
1 garlic clove, crushed
300g (9½oz) Swiss brown mushrooms
1 tablespoon fresh flat-leaf parsley leaves, chopped
Sea salt and freshly cracked black pepper to taste
1 tablespoon olive oil, extra
250g (8 oz) baby English spinach leaves

Heat butter and oil in a frying pan; add mushrooms and garlic and stir-fry for 6 minutes or until cooked through. Season and stir through parsley.

For the spinach, heat extra oil in a large frying pan, add the spinach and stir-fry for 2 minutes or until spinach has just wilted. Season spinach then serve onto plates topped with the mushrooms.

Total cooking time: 5 minutes preparation, 8 minutes cooking
Serves: 2

SNACKS AND SIDE-DISHES

Cheese and sliced/cured meats

Fruit

Fresh vegetables

Nuts

Salad of rocket with walnuts and feta

Asian salad

Roast vegetables

Tomato and basil salad

Salsa verde salad

Cucumber and caper salad

Roasted red onions and Roma tomatoes

Simple rocket salad

Tomato salsa

Salad with feta, cherry tomatoes and cucumber

Barbecued vegetables

Greek salad

Cheese and sliced/cured meats
Protein

Cheese is classified as a protein. You can eat cheese with any protein meal and between protein meals, such as for morning or afternoon tea. The only cheese not suitable is any cheese made with goat's milk or any cheese containing fruit, nuts or poppy seeds. You should also eat soft white cheeses in moderation and use mascarpone cheese with caution. You are free to enjoy hard yellow cheese.

Sliced/cured meats are also a good snack which can be eaten with cheese. You can eat meats with any protein meal or between protein meals. Some sliced/cured meats will have sugar as an ingredient on the packaging – this is because the meat is cured using a mixture of sugar and salt. You will notice that sugar features low on the list of ingredients. You can still eat this meat as a protein. Other sliced/cured meats use sugar as an ingredient mixed with the meat product during processing; these may cause your weight loss to plateau. When selecting sliced/cured meat you should read the nutritional panel on the product – you should look for a sugar content of less than 1g per 100g serving. If you are unsure, or you have reached a plateau in your weight loss, then try leaving the sliced/cured meat out of your diet.

An example of a serve of cheese:
- 2 slices of cheddar cheese

Examples of serves of sliced or cured meat:
- 1 slice of roasted turkey breast *or*
- 3 slices of pepperoni

Fruit
Carbohydrate

Fruit is generally a moderate carbohydrate and therefore should be eaten in moderation. Remember to observe the time intervals between eating a carbohydrate meal and a protein meal when eating fruit.

Fruit that can be eaten in moderation include:

- Apples
- Dried apples
- Oranges
- Grapefruit
- Apricots
- Dried apricots
- Cherries
- Peaches
- Pears
- Plums
- Rhubarb
- Strawberries

Fruit that you should avoid include:

- Bananas
- Kiwi fruit
- Mango
- Paw paw
- Pineapple
- Rockmelon
- Watermelon
- Raisins
- Sultanas
- Currants

- Grapes
- Figs
- Dates

Examples of serves of fruit include:

- 1 handful of dried apricots *or*
- 140g (4½oz) of diced pears in natural juice *or*
- 1 orange *or*
- 6 strawberries

Fresh vegetables
Carbohydrate/Protein

You can make a quick and easy low GI snack using good carbo-hydrate vegetables. These vegetables will have a GI of less than 20 and can be eaten with either protein or carbohydrate style meals or between meals. Fresh vegetables are a good source of fibre and nutrients. Fresh vegetables that you can eat include:

- Tomato
- Celery
- Cucumber
- Mushroom
- Capsicum
- Zucchini
- Fennel

You can eat fresh vegetables served with the suggested dips in this recipe section.

Nuts
Protein

The following nuts have a GI of zero (or an undetectable GI) – they are therefore classified as a Protein meal. These nuts are pecans, walnuts, Brazil nuts, macadamias, almonds and hazelnuts. Although these nuts have a zero GI some people have found that they reached a plateau in their weight loss when eating too many nuts, particularly when eating macadamias and almonds. If you find your weight loss plateaus when including these nuts in your diet, then either decrease the quantity you are eating or remove them from your diet. We recommend no more than 5–6 nuts as an individual snack serving once per day.

Salad of rocket with walnuts and feta

Protein

Using good quality ingredients makes this very simple salad taste wonderful – you can even substitute the olive oil with walnut oil if you have some handy. Walnuts have been shown to improve heart health as they are packed with good fats called omega-6 and omega-3 fatty acids.

2 cups rocket leaves

50g (1½oz) feta cheese, crumbled

2 tablespoons walnut pieces

1 tablespoon olive oil

Combine all ingredients and serve as a side-salad.

Total cooking time: 5 minutes preparation
Serves: 2 side-dish servings

Asian salad

Carbohydrate/Protein

If you are unable to find Thai basil you can substitute it with ordinary English basil.

2 cups mixed salad leaves

¼ continental cucumber, sliced

¼ cup fresh Thai basil leaves, chopped

2 tablespoons Vietnamese mint, chopped

¼ long red chilli, seeded and chopped

¼ red capsicum, seeded and thinly sliced

2 teaspoons lime juice

2 teaspoons white wine vinegar

Combine all ingredients, toss well and serve as a side-dish to carbohydrate or protein style meals.

Total cooking time: 5 minutes preparation
Serves: 2 side-dish servings

Roast vegetables

Protein

Lebanese eggplants, used in this recipe, are the long thin-shaped eggplants. You should easily be able to find them at your local supermarket or fruit and vegetable store.

½ red onion, end left intact, cut into wedges

6 asparagus spears, trimmed

2 Lebanese eggplants, halved lengthways

1 baby yellow squash, quartered

1 Roma tomato, halved

1 zucchini, halved lengthways, then quartered

4 tablespoons olive oil

1 teaspoon dried oregano

Sea salt and freshly cracked black pepper to taste

50g (1½oz) feta, crumbled

¼ cup fresh flat-leaf parsley leaves, chopped

In a bowl combine onion, asparagus, eggplant, squash, tomato, zucchini, oil, oregano and seasoning. Toss together well to coat vegetables in oil, oregano and seasoning. Arrange vegetables on a baking tray and cook at 180°C (350°F) for 1 hour. Remove from oven and serve onto plates, scatter over feta cheese and parsley. Serve as a protein-style side-dish.

Total cooking time: 10 minutes preparation, 1 hour cooking
Serves: 2

Tomato and basil salad
Protein

50g (1½oz) baby English spinach leaves

1 tomato cut into 8 wedges

2 tablespoons olive oil

1 tablespoon white wine vinegar

10 fresh basil leaves

Sea salt and freshly cracked black pepper to taste

For the salad, arrange spinach leaves onto two plates, top with tomato wedges, drizzle over the olive oil and vinegar and scatter over the basil and season.

Total cooking time: 5 minutes preparation
Serves: 2

Salsa verde salad

Protein

2 canned anchovies, mashed

1 tablespoons white wine vinegar

2 tablespoons olive oil

1 tomato, seeded and chopped

¼ cup fresh flat-leaf parsley leaves, finely chopped

2 cups mixed salad leaves

½ Lebanese cucumber, sliced

Sea salt and freshly cracked black pepper to taste

Combine anchovies, vinegar and olive oil together; mix well. Combine all other ingredients; drizzle over anchovy mixture and toss salad well to combine. Serve as a protein-style side-dish.

Total cooking time: 5 minutes preparation
Serves: 2 side-dish servings

Cucumber and caper salad

Protein

2 Lebanese cucumbers, halved, seeded and chopped

Juice of ½ lemon

2 tablespoons olive oil

2 tablespoons fresh flat-leaf parsley, chopped

1 tablespoon baby capers

Sea salt and freshly ground black pepper to taste

Combine all ingredients and toss well. Serve as a side-dish.

Total cooking time: 5 minutes preparation
Serves: 2

Roasted red onions and Roma tomatoes

Protein

½ red onion, peeled, ends left intact, cut into wedges

2 Roma tomatoes, halved lengthways

2 tablespoon olive oil

1 teaspoon dried oregano

Sea salt and freshly cracked black pepper to taste

Arrange onion and tomato on a baking tray; drizzle with oil and scatter over oregano and seasoning. Roast at 180°C (350°F) for 45 minutes. Serve as a side-dish.

Total cooking time: 5 minutes preparation, 45 minutes cooking
Serves: 2

Simple rocket salad
Protein

Rocket is a salad leaf with a peppery and slightly bitter taste. It is also known by the names arugula and Italian cress. If you are unable to find rocket leaves or you don't like the taste then you can substitute with another type of salad leaf such as baby spinach leaves or baby mesclun salad mix.

2 cups rocket leaves

Juice of ½ lemon

1 tablespoon olive oil

Sea salt and freshly cracked black pepper to taste

Combine all ingredients, toss well and serve as a side dish.

Total cooking time: 5 minutes preparation
Serves: 2

Tomato salsa

Carbohydrate/Protein

¼ red onion, very finely chopped

½ garlic clove, crushed

½ fresh long red chilli, seeded and finely chopped

4 Roma tomatoes, seeded and finely chopped

¼ cup fresh coriander, chopped

Juice of ½ lime

Sea salt and freshly ground black pepper to taste

Combine all ingredients; mix well and serve as a side dish.

Total cooking time: 5 minutes preparation
Serves: 2

Salad with feta, cherry tomatoes and cucumber

Protein

2 cups mixed salad leaves

50g (1½oz) feta cheese, crumbled

8 cherry tomatoes, halved

½ Lebanese cucumber, sliced

1 tablespoon lemon juice

1 tablespoon olive oil

Sea salt and freshly cracked black pepper to taste

Combine all ingredients, toss well and serve as a side dish.

Total cooking time: 5 minutes preparation
Serves: 2

Barbecued vegetables

Protein

1 zucchini, sliced 1 cm (½ inch) thick lengthways

1 baby yellow squash, sliced 1 cm (½ inch) thick

4 asparagus spears, trimmed

2 Lebanese eggplants, halved lengthways

½ cup olive oil

2 tablespoons fresh flat-leaf parsley leaves

1 teaspoon dried oregano

1 garlic clove, crushed

Sea salt and freshly cracked black pepper to taste

Combine all ingredients together and toss well. Cook vegetables on a heated oiled barbecue for approximately 8 minutes each side or until browned and tender. Baste with any remaining olive oil while cooking. Serve as a protein-style side-dish.

Total cooking time: 10 minutes preparation, 16 minutes cooking
Serves: 2

Greek salad
Protein

¼ red onion

2 tomatoes, seeded and chopped

½ cucumber, sliced

50g (1½oz) feta

2 tablespoons fresh basil leaves, torn

1 tablespoon olive oil

1 tablespoon lemon juice

Combine all ingredients together; toss well.

Total cooking time: 5 minutes preparation
Serves: 2

MAINS

Spicy vegetable soup with red kidney beans and coriander

Moussaka

Salad with sardine fillets

Lamb stir-fry

Tofu balls with tamarind and tomato sauce

Barbecued haloumi and vegetables with lemon and capers

Chicken burgers

Roast pork

Stir-fried seafood

Chicken soup

Vegetable salad

Cajun beef stir-fry

Fresh pasta with passata, capers and parsley

Barbecued lamb cutlets

Frittata with bacon and sun-dried tomatoes

Mushroom risotto

Middle Eastern burgers

Chicken and pecan salad with lemon aioli

Beef round medallions

Salmon muffins

Basmati rice salad with tomatoes, fennel and fresh herbs

Asian pork stir-fry

Egg roll-ups

Roast lamb

Barbecued fish fillets

Vegetable kebabs

Spicy chicken Stir-fry

Spinach and ricotta tarts

Spicy vegetable soup with red kidney beans and coriander

Carbohydrate

Red kidney beans are an excellent source of iron, magnesium and folate, giving more than 20 per cent of the recommended daily intake of these nutrients.

When following the meals planner this recipe makes enough for 2 people for 3 serves each. Keep frozen in micro-wave- and freezer-proof containers in 6 individual serves. To reheat when defrosted, place in the microwave for 5 minutes on high.

2 onions, sliced

3 garlic cloves, crushed

2 long red chillies, seeded and chopped, or to taste

2 celery sticks, sliced

2 zucchinis, sliced

4 baby yellow squash, sliced

800g (28oz) diced tomatoes

6 cups vegetable stock

2 medium sweet potatoes, peeled and diced

400g (14oz) red kidney beans

1 teaspoon turmeric

½ teaspoon paprika

½ teaspoon ground coriander

½ cup fresh coriander leaves, chopped

Sea salt and freshly cracked black pepper to taste

In a large saucepan combine onion, garlic, chilli, celery, zucchini, squash, tomatoes, stock and potato. Cover, bring to the boil, then

reduce heat and allow to simmer for 20 minutes. Add kidney beans,
turmeric, paprika, ground coriander and continue to simmer for a
further 15 minutes. Stir through coriander leaves and seasoning
and serve.

Total cooking time: 10 minutes preparation, 40 minutes cooking
Serves: 6

Moussaka

Protein

Moussaka is a traditional Greek dish. It is made with a layer of fried eggplant followed by layer of meat sauce and topped with a white sauce. The white sauce topping, which usually contains high GI carbohydrates, has been substituted with tasty cheese and Parmesan cheese for this recipe.

When following the meal planner this recipe makes enough for 2 people for three servings each. Once cooked, allow moussaka to cool slightly then cut into 6 pieces and place into individual freezer- and microwave-proof containers and freeze. For reheating defrosted servings of moussaka, place in the microwave for 6 minutes on high.

2 medium eggplants, peeled and sliced lengthways
  1 cm (½ inch) thick
¼ cup olive oil, heated
Sea salt and freshly ground black pepper
2 tablespoons olive oil, extra
2 large garlic cloves, minced
1 medium onion, minced
500g (16oz) lean beef mince
400g (14oz) diced tomatoes
2 tablespoons tomato paste
1 teaspoon ground allspice
½ teaspoon cinnamon
200g (7oz) grated tasty cheese
½ cup grated Parmesan cheese

Sprinkle eggplant slices liberally with salt and allow to stand 2 hours before rinsing and patting dry. Heat a large frying pan and add a little of the olive oil, place eggplant slices in the frying pan in batches, season with salt and pepper, and fry 3 minutes each side until browned, basting regularly with olive oil. Place eggplant on absorbent paper to drain.

For the beef mixture, heat the extra olive oil in a large frying pan, add onion and garlic and stir-fry 5 minutes until onion has softened. Add the mince to the onion mixture and stir-fry until browned. Add all other ingredients and simmer for 20 minutes until juices have condensed; season.

In a casserole dish layer eggplant slices, top with the beef mixture, scatter over the cheeses. Bake in oven at 200°C (390°F) for 30 minutes or until cheese is golden brown.

Total cooking time: 10 minutes preparation, 2 hours standing, 1 hour cooking
Serves: 6

Salad with sardine fillets

Protein

Sardines are packed full of important nutrients such as omega-3 fatty acids, protein and calcium, and are rich in phosphorus, iron, potassium, vitamin B6 and niacin.

200g (7oz) sardine fillets in oil

Juice of ½ lemon

2 tablespoons red wine vinegar

2 tablespoons fresh flat-leaf parsley leaves, chopped

1 tablespoon fresh thyme leaves, chopped

1 garlic clove, crushed

Sea salt and freshly cracked black pepper to taste

1 Lebanese cucumber, sliced

10 cherry tomatoes, halved

3 cups mixed lettuce leaves

Combine sardines and oil with the lemon juice, vinegar, parsley, thyme, garlic and seasoning. Marinate for 1 hour in the refrigerator.

Toss together the cucumber, tomatoes and mixed lettuce leaves, then divide between two plates. Top the lettuce leaves with the marinated sardines and drizzle over the marinade.

Total cooking time: 10 minutes preparation, 1 hour marinating
Serves: 2

Lamb stir-fry

Protein

1 tablespoon oil

1 onion, sliced

300g (9½oz) diced lamb

½ stick celery, thinly sliced

100g (3½oz) green beans, trimmed and cut into 5cm
 (2 inch) lengths

2 tomatoes, cut into wedges

¼ cup fresh flat-leaf parsley leaves, chopped

Sea salt and freshly cracked black pepper to taste

Heat oil in a large saucepan, add onion and garlic and cook until onion softens. Add lamb and stir-fry 5 minutes over high heat or until meat is browned all over. Add celery and beans and stir-fry a further 5 minutes. Add tomatoes and cook 1 minute. Stir through parsley and seasoning and serve.

Total cooking time: 5 minutes preparation, 15 minutes cooking
Serves: 2

Tofu balls with tamarind and tomato sauce

Carbohydrate

Use calcium fortified tofu if it is available at your supermarket or maybe at your local health food store.

When following the meal planner this recipe makes 32 tofu balls for 5 serves per person for 2 lunches and 3 per person for 2 snacks. Tofu balls should be frozen with plastic separating them so you can easily remove the quantity you require to defrost for lunches and snacks. The tamarind and tomato sauce can be kept in the refrigerator in a sealed container. Serve the tofu balls and the sauce either cold or hot. For reheating tofu balls, place in the microwave for 2 minutes on high. For reheating tamarind and tomato sauce, place the required amount of sauce in the microwave for 20–30 seconds.

400g (14oz) hard tofu, roughly chopped
1 garlic clove, crushed
¼ cup fresh coriander leaves
2 tablespoons fresh Vietnamese mint leaves
1 teaspoon tamarind puree
¼ teaspoon chilli powder, or to taste
½ teaspoon salt

Tamarind and tomato sauce
1 spring onion, sliced
1 long red chilli, seeded and chopped
2 Roma tomatoes, seeded and chopped
½ teaspoon tamarind puree
Sea salt and freshly cracked black pepper to taste

In a blender combine tofu, garlic, coriander, mint, tamarind, chilli and salt. Process to form a smooth paste. Roll paste into 32 balls. Place on a non-stick baking tray and bake at 180°C (350°F) for 30 minutes.

For the tamarind and tomato sauce, process all ingredients and serve over the tofu balls or separately as a dipping sauce. The sauce can also be heated before serving if required.

Serve tofu balls as an entrée or as a main dish with a suitable protein style side-dish.

Total cooking time: 10 minutes preparation, 30 minutes cooking
Makes: 32

Barbecued haloumi and vegetables with lemon and capers

Protein

1 red capsicum, seeded and quartered

½ cup olive oil

1 garlic clove, crushed

Sea salt and freshly cracked black pepper

1 tablespoon mixed dried herbs

2 Lebanese eggplants, halved lengthways

6 asparagus spears, trimmed

1 zucchini, trimmed then sliced 1 cm (½ inch) thick
  lengthways

½ red onion, ends intact, cut into wedges

2 baby yellow squash, sliced 1 cm (½ inch) thick

100g (3½oz) haloumi, sliced 1 cm (½ inch) thick

1 teaspoon lemon juice

1 teaspoon baby capers

1 tablespoon fresh flat-leaf parsley

Place capsicum under a hot grill, skin side up, until skin blackens and blisters. Allow to cool in a plastic bag before peeling.

Combine olive oil, garlic, seasoning and mixed herbs. Baste eggplant, asparagus, zucchini, onion, squash and haloumi. Cook vegetables and haloumi on a heated oiled barbecue hotplate for 8 minutes each side or until browned and cooked through; baste regularly with any remaining garlic and olive oil mixture.

Arrange vegetables and haloumi onto two plates; drizzle over lemon juice and scatter over capers and parsley, then serve.

Total cooking time: 10 minutes preparation, 16 minutes cooking
Serves: 2

Chicken burgers

Protein

When following the meal planner this recipe makes enough chicken burgers for 2 people for 2 lunches each. Once cooked, allow the chicken burgers to cool slightly before placing into a container for freezing. Freeze until ready to use. To reheat defrosted 4 piece servings of chicken burgers, place in the microwave for 3 minutes on high.

500g (16oz) chicken mince
½ small brown onion, minced
4 tablespoons fresh flat-leaf parsley leaves
2 egg whites, lightly beaten
½ teaspoon sea salt
Dash of pepper

For the burgers, combine all ingredients. Divide mixture into burgers. Cook burgers on a preheated barbecue 3–4 minutes each side or until golden brown and cooked through. Serve with a suitable protein-style side-dish.

Total cooking time: 15 minutes
Makes: 16 burgers

Roast pork
Protein

750g (24oz) boned pork loin roll
4 tablespoons olive oil
Sea salt

Dry the pork skin well with absorbent paper. Cut cross hatches through the pork skin to the fat beneath. Rub olive oil and liberal amounts of salt into the pork skin. Place pork on a baking tray, skin side up. Roast at 220°C (425°F) for 10 minutes then reduce heat and roast at 180°C (350°F) for 50 minutes or until juices run clear. Stand in a warm place for 10 minutes before carving. Serve in slices with an appropriate protein-style side dish.

Total cooking time: 5 minutes preparation, 1 hour cooking,
10 minutes standing
Serves: 2

Stir-fried seafood

Protein

1 tablespoon olive oil

½ red onion, finely chopped

1 garlic clove, crushed

1 squid hood, scored and sliced lengthways into 2 cm
 (1 inch) wide pieces

2 baby octopus, quartered

100g (3½oz) prawn meat

1 white fish fillet, diced

2 tablespoons fresh flat-leaf parsley leaves, chopped

Sea salt and freshly cracked black pepper, to taste

Heat oil in a large wok, add onion and garlic and cook until onion softens. Add squid, octopus, prawns and fish; stir-fry for 3 minutes or until seafood is tender and cooked through. Stir through parsley and seasoning and serve.

Total cooking time: 5 minutes preparation, 5 minutes cooking
Serves: 2

Chicken soup

Protein

1 tablespoon olive oil

2 chicken breast fillets

1 tablespoon olive oil, extra

½ onion, finely chopped

½ garlic clove, crushed

½ stick of celery, finely sliced

1 teaspoon freshly grated ginger

4 cups hot water

2 egg whites, lightly beaten

1 tablespoon fresh flat-leaf parsley, chopped

Sea salt and freshly cracked black pepper, to taste

Heat oil in a frying pan, add the chicken fillets and cook for
4 minutes each side or until browned and cooked through. Set chicken
aside; allow to rest for 5 minutes before shredding meat.

To the frying pan add extra olive oil, onion and garlic and cook
until onion softens. Add celery and ginger and cook a further
5 minutes. Add water and shredded chicken, then heat. Stir through
egg whites, parsley and seasoning and serve.

Total cooking time: 20 minutes
Serves: 2

Vegetable salad
Carbohydrate

1 small red onion, skin removed, ends left intact, cut into
 wedges

1 small zucchini, trimmed and quartered

6 button mushrooms, peeled, stalks removed

1 baby yellow squash, trimmed and quartered

2 Lebanese eggplants, halved lengthways

4 tablespoons olive oil

Sea salt and freshly cracked black pepper to taste

1 tablespoon dried oregano

1 red capsicum, seeded and quartered

2 canned artichoke hearts, quartered

½ head broccoli, divided into florets

Salt and pepper to taste

*Mix together onion, zucchini, mushrooms, squash, eggplant, oil,
herbs and seasoning. Toss together well to coat vegetables in the oil,
oregano and seasoning. Place vegetables on a baking tray and cook at
180°C (350°F) for 1 hour. Remove from oven and allow to cool.*

*Grill capsicum until skin is blackened and blistered. Allow to cool
then remove skin and slice into strips lengthways.*

*Steam broccoli florets 3 minutes or until tender so they retain their
crispness and color. Combine all vegetables; arrange onto two plates.
Serve topped with tomato salsa.*

Total cooking time: 10 minutes preparation, 1 hour cooking
Serves: 2

Cajun beef stir-fry
Protein

You can purchase Cajun seasoning in the dried herbs and spices section of the supermarket. Make sure that it does not contained added sugar as an ingredient.

1 tablespoon olive oil

1 brown onion, sliced

1 garlic clove, crushed

450g (15oz) lean beef, thinly sliced

1 teaspoon Cajun seasoning

100g (3½oz) green beans, trimmed and cut into 5 cm (2 inch) lengths

½ head of broccoli, cut into florets

¼ cup fresh flat-leaf parsley, chopped

Sea salt and freshly cracked black pepper to taste

Heat oil in a large wok, add onion and garlic and stir-fry until onion softens. Add beef and stir-fry for 4 minutes or until browned. Add beans and broccoli and stir-fry for 5 minutes or until vegetables are tender and cooked through. Stir through parsley and seasoning and serve.

Total cooking time: 5 minutes preparation, 10 minutes cooking
Serves: 2

Fresh pasta with passata, capers and parsley

Carbohydrate

Tomato passata is pureed tomatoes found in the pasta sauce and tomato paste section of the supermarket.

300g (9½oz) fresh fettuccine pasta

1 cup tomato passata

2 tablespoons red wine vinegar

2 teaspoons baby capers

¼ cup fresh flat-leaf parsley leaves, chopped

Sea salt and freshly cracked black pepper to taste

Cook pasta in a saucepan of boiling salted water for 3 minutes; drain. Heat tomato passata in a large saucepan, add the pasta, vinegar, capers, parsley and seasoning; toss well to combine and serve.

Total cooking time: 5 minutes preparation, 5 minutes cooking
Serves: 2

Barbecued lamb cutlets

Protein

6 lamb cutlets

Sea salt and freshly cracked black pepper

*On a heated oiled barbecue cook lamb cutlets for 2–3 minutes each
side or until browned and cooked through. Season with salt and
pepper and serve with appropriate protein-style barbecued vegetables
or other protein-style side-dish.*

Total cooking time: 6 minutes
Serves: 2

Frittata with bacon and sun-dried tomatoes

Protein

When using the meal planner this recipe will make enough for 2 people for 2 serves each. You should freeze the frittata in microwave- and freezer-proof containers in 4 single serve portions. For re-heating when defrosted, place in the microwave for 6 minutes on high.

1 tablespoon olive oil

1 red onion, finely chopped

1 garlic clove, crushed

2 rindless bacon rashers, chopped

6 button mushrooms, sliced

8 semi sun-dried tomatoes, sliced

100g (3½oz) green beans, trimmed and cut into 5 cm
 (2 inch) lengths

300g (10oz) baby English spinach leaves

8 eggs, lightly beaten

½ cup fresh flat-leaf parsley leaves, chopped

Sea salt and freshly cracked black pepper to taste

1 cup grated cheese

¼ cup grated Parmesan cheese

Heat oil in a large frying pan, add onion and garlic and cook until onion softens. Add bacon and mushrooms and stir-fry for 5 minutes. Add tomatoes, beans and spinach leaves and stir-fry for a further 5 minutes.

Combine eggs, parsley and seasoning. Add cooked vegetables and bacon to the egg mixture and combine well. Pour mixture into a

square casserole dish and bake at 180°C (350°F) for 40 minutes.
Serve in slices with an appropriate protein-style side-dish.

Total cooking time: 10 minutes preparation, 50 minutes cooking
Serves: 4

Mushroom risotto
Carbohydrate

You can use different types of mushroom varieties to make this recipe, so if you can't find some of the suggested mushrooms in the ingredients list, then just substitute for what is available at your fruit and vegetable store.

When following the meal planner this recipe makes enough for 2 people for 2 meals each. Divide into 4 freezer-proof containers and freeze. To reheat defrosted individual servings, place in the microwave for 3 minutes on high, stir once during heating.

4 spring onions, sliced
1 garlic clove, crushed
2 teaspoons freshly-grated ginger
8 oyster mushrooms
6 Swiss brown mushrooms, quartered
4 button mushrooms, sliced
190g (6oz) whole champignons, drained
½ teaspoon cinnamon
2 cups basmati rice
7 cups vegetable stock
¾ cup fresh coriander leaves, chopped
Sea salt and freshly cracked black pepper to taste

In a large wok stir-fry onions and garlic with ¼ cup of water until onions soften. Add ginger and mushrooms and another ¼ cup of water and stir-fry for 4 minutes. Add cinnamon and basmati rice and stir-fry for 3 minutes. Add 1 cup of stock and cook over low heat until liquid is absorbed. Repeat adding the rest of the stock

1 cup at a time until rice is soft and cooked through. Stir through coriander and seasoning and serve.

Total cooking time: 5 minutes preparation, 30 minutes cooking
Serves: 4

Middle Eastern burgers
Protein

250g (8oz) mince beef

¼ teaspoon chilli powder

2 teaspoons ground cumin

½ teaspoon ground coriander

½ teaspoon salt

¼ teaspoon ground black pepper

1 egg white, lightly beaten

Combine all ingredients together; mix well then form into burgers. Cook burgers in a frying pan or on a barbecue plate for 3 minutes each side or until browned and cooked through. Serve burgers with an appropriate protein-style side-dish.

Total cooking time: 5 minutes preparation, 6 minutes cooking
Serves: 2

Chicken and pecan salad with lemon aioli

Protein

Pecans are a good source of fibre and contain over 19 vitamins and minerals; including vitamin A, vitamin E, folic acid, calcium, magnesium, phosphorus, potassium, several B vitamins and zinc. Research has shown that pecans can contribute to lowering cholesterol levels when included in a healthy diet.

1 tablespoon olive oil

2 chicken breast fillets

4 cups mixed salad leaves

20g (½oz) pecans

50g (1½oz) feta cheese, crumbled

½ Lebanese cucumber, sliced

10 cherry tomatoes, halved

1 tablespoon fresh mint leaves, chopped

Sea salt and freshly cracked black pepper, to taste

Lemon aioli

1 egg yolk

1 teaspoon lemon juice

¼ cup olive oil

Sea salt and freshly ground black pepper, to taste

Heat oil in a large frying pan, cook chicken 3–4 minutes each side or until golden brown and cooked through. Allow chicken to rest 5 minutes before slicing. Combine chicken, salad leaves, pecans, feta, cucumber, tomato, mint and seasoning and toss well.

For the aioli, combine egg yolks and lemon juice. Gradually add oil until well combined and sauce thickens. Season, then pour over the salad. Toss well to coat salad in the aioli, then serve.

Total cooking time: 5 minutes preparation, 8 minutes cooking
Serves: 2

Beef round medallions
Protein

2 beef round medallions
1 anchovy, mashed
1 tablespoon olive oil
Dash of pepper

Combine anchovy, olive oil and pepper. Baste beef medallions with the olive oil mixture; wrap in plastic and refrigerate for 30 minutes. Cook beef on a heated oiled barbecue for 3–4 minutes each side or until browned and cooked to your liking. Serve with an appropriate protein-style side-dish.

Total cooking time: 5 minutes preparation, 30 minutes marinating, 8 minutes cooking
Serves: 2

Salmon muffins
Protein

Canned salmon, with the bones, is an excellent source of calcium; 100g (3½oz) of canned salmon provides 15% of your daily recommended intake of calcium.

When following the meal planner this recipe makes enough salmon muffins for 2 people for 1 dinner and 1 snack each. Once cooked, allow the salmon muffins to cool slightly before placing into a container for freezing. Freeze until ready to use. To reheat when defrosted, place in the microwave for 2 minutes on high. To reheat when frozen, place in the microwave for 6 minutes on high.

415g (14oz) salmon and bones, drained
6 eggs
4 tablespoons fresh mascarpone cheese
½ cup fresh dill
¼ cup fresh tarragon
Sea salt and freshly cracked black pepper to taste

Combine all ingredients together in a food processor and blend until well combined. Pour mixture into muffin tins and bake at 180°C (350°F) for 35 minutes or until firm to the touch and golden brown.

Total cooking time: 5 minutes preparation, 35 minutes cooking
Makes: 16 muffins

Basmati rice salad with tomatoes, fennel and fresh herbs

Carbohydrate

Fennel is a white-coloured, aniseed-tasting vegetable. Reserve the frond from the tops of the baby fennel for use in this recipe. If you cannot find baby fennel you can use ½ a fennel bulb instead, or if you have no luck with this, then just substitute it for 1 Lebanese cucumber halved, seeded and diced.

When following the meal planner this recipe makes enough for 2 people for 2 meals each. You should keep it refrigerated.

1¼ cups basmati rice
½ red onion, thinly sliced
4 Roma tomatoes, seeded and chopped
2 baby fennel bulb, trimmed, halved and thinly sliced
2 tablespoons white wine vinegar
Juice of ½ lemon
½ cup fresh flat-leaf parsley leaves, chopped
¼ cup fresh basil leaves, chopped
¼ cup baby fennel fronds, chopped
Sea salt and freshly cracked black pepper to taste

Cook the rice in the usual method. Rinse with cold water and drain well. Combine rice with all other ingredients and serve.

Total cooking time: 5 minutes preparation, 25 minutes cooking
Serves: 4

Asian pork stir-fry

Protein

1 tablespoon peanut oil

1 teaspoon sesame oil

2 spring onions, sliced

400g (14oz) diced pork

1 star anise

1 cinnamon stick

2 cloves

1 slice ginger

4 button mushrooms, sliced

3 cups wom bok

2 cups bean shoots

Sea salt and freshly cracked black pepper to taste

Heat oils in a large wok, add onion and garlic and stir-fry
2 minutes. Add pork, star anise, cinnamon, cloves and ginger, then
stir-fry 4 minutes or until pork is golden brown. Add mushrooms
and stir-fry a further 2 minutes. Add the wom bok and bean shoots
and fry 3 minutes. Season and serve.

Total cooking time: 5 minutes preparation, 15 minutes cooking
Serves: 2

Egg roll-ups
Protein

Olive oil

5 eggs, lightly beaten

2 cups rocket leaves

60g (2oz) feta, crumbled

4 slices of prosciutto

8 semi sun-dried tomatoes, thinly sliced

8 fresh basil leaves

1 tablespoon olive oil, extra

1 teaspoon lemon juice

Sea salt and freshly cracked black pepper to taste

Heat a little oil in a large frying pan. Pour a quarter of the beaten egg mixture into the pan and cook for 2 minutes or until set. Repeat with remaining mixture. Place each egg crepe on a plate, then top with rocket, feta, prosciutto, tomato and basil. Drizzle over oil and lemon juice and season. Roll up the crepes and serve.

Total cooking time: 10 minutes preparation, 15 minutes cooking
Serves: 2

Roast lamb

Protein

¼ cup olive oil

3 garlic cloves, crushed

Zest of 1 lemon

1 tablespoon baby capers, chopped

2 tablespoons fresh thyme leaves, chopped

½ teaspoon sea salt

¼ teaspoon freshly cracked black pepper

700g (23oz) boneless lamb leg roast, tied in a roll

Combine oil, garlic, zest, capers, thyme, salt and pepper in a mortar and pestle and crush to form a coarse paste. Rub paste into the lamb. Place lamb on a baking tray and bake at 160°C (320°F) for 55 minutes or until juices run clear. Once cooked allow to rest in a warm place for 10 minutes before carving. Serve in slices with protein style roast vegetables or another appropriate protein style side-dish.

Total cooking time: 5 minutes preparation, 55 minutes cooking, 10 minutes standing
Serves: 2

Barbecued fish fillets
Protein

2 large white fish fillets of choice

Zest of ½ lemon

Sea salt and freshly cracked black pepper

1 tablespoon olive oil

Lemon wedges to serve

Rub fish fillets all over with the oil, zest and seasoning. Cook fish on a heated oiled barbecue plate for 3 minutes each side or until cooked through. Serve with an appropriate protein-style side-dish and lemon wedges.

Total cooking time: 5 minutes preparation, 6 minutes cooking
Serves: 2

Vegetable kebabs
Protein

People often ask why this dish is classed as a protein-style meal when it is made from vegetables which are carbohydrates. The reason is the use of olive oil to baste the vegetables. Olive oil is used for ease of cooking and for flavour. If you decide to grill these kebabs and not use the olive oil then this would make this dish suitable as either a protein or carbohydrate-style meal.

6 bamboo skewers, pre-soaked

12 button mushrooms

1 red capsicum, seeded and cut into 5 cm (2 inch) pieces

6 small shallots, peeled, ends left intact

6 canned artichoke hearts, halved

2 baby yellow squash, cut into wedges

2 tablespoons olive oil

1 teaspoon mixed dried herbs

Sea salt and freshly cracked black pepper to taste

Thread alternating vegetables onto the skewers. Brush vegetables with oil, scatter over herbs and season. Cook vegetable skewers on a barbecue for 10 minutes; turn several times during cooking. Serve with an appropriate protein-style side-dish.

Total cooking time: 10 minutes preparation, 10 minutes cooking
Serves: 2

Spicy chicken stir-fry

Protein

Sambal oelek is an Indonesian-style hot chilli paste. Make sure that the brand you purchase does not contain added sugar as an ingredient. If you are unable to purchase sambal oelek, then substitute with ¼ teaspoon of chilli powder or to your taste.

1 tablespoon peanut oil

1 teaspoon sesame oil

1 onion, sliced

1 garlic clove, crushed

350g (12oz) chicken mince

2 teaspoons cumin

½ teaspoon sambal oelek, or to taste

2 cups wom bok, shredded

100g (3½oz) green beans, cut into 5 cm (2 inch) lengths

1 stick of celery

3 tomatoes, chopped

Juice of ½ lemon

3 tablespoons fresh flat-leaf parsley leaves, chopped

Sea salt and freshly cracked black pepper to taste

Heat oils in a large wok, add onion and garlic and cook until onion softens. Add chicken mince and stir-fry for 5 minutes or until browned. Add the cumin, sambal oelek, wom bok, green beans, celery and tomatoes, then stir-fry for 5 minutes. Add the lemon juice, parsley and seasoning; stir through then serve.

Total cooking time: 5 minutes preparation, 10 minutes cooking
Serves: 2–3

Spinach and ricotta tarts
Protein

When following the meal planner this recipe makes enough for 2 people for 2 meals each. The recipe makes 16 tarts in total, 4 for each meal. Freeze the tarts in a freezer-proof container with plastic wrap between them for ease of separation. Serve hot or cold. To reheat serves of 4 defrosted tarts, place in the microwave for 2 minutes on high.

500g (17oz) fresh ricotta
¾ cup mozzarella cheese, grated
¼ cup Parmesan cheese, grated
250g (8oz) packet frozen spinach, thawed and squeezed of excess fluid
10 sun-dried tomatoes, chopped
¼ cup fresh flat-leaf parsley, chopped
2 eggs, lightly beaten
Sea salt and freshly cracked black pepper, to taste

Combine all ingredients together. Spoon into greased muffin tins and bake at 180°C (350°F) for 30 minutes. Serve with appropriate protein-style side-dish.

Total cooking time: 5 minutes preparation, 30 minutes cooking
Makes: 16 tarts

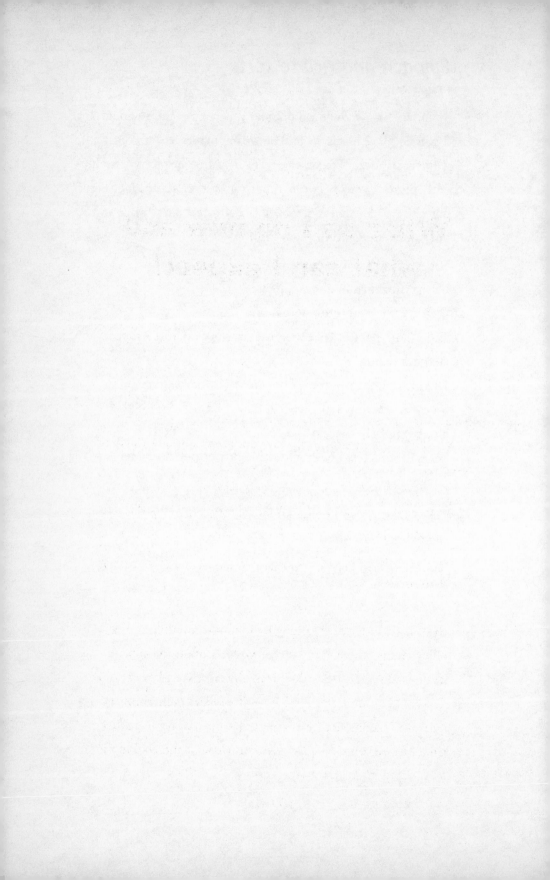

CHAPTER 2

What do I do now and what can I expect?

Back to me again, "Dr John" your narrator.

There are three things that you must do to get the best results.

1. **Throw out all the bad carbs in the house:** This way you are not tempted by the sight of foods you shouldn't be eating. If you can't bring yourself to put it in the bin, give it to someone outside of the home.

2. **Prepare food in advance:** I cannot over-emphasise this point enough. It is critical that you maintain the continuity to achieve the best results. In a perfect world we would just whiz around the kitchen and prepare something for ourselves before sitting down and enjoying it. In reality, time is something we have precious little of and cooking is

not something that many of us can devote ourselves to on a daily basis, so you have to set aside at least a few hours each week to prepare some of the dishes. What Chérie and I do is spend one morning or a few hours in the afternoon, usually on the weekend, cooking up usually three of the dishes. We do it on a big scale, like a moussaka the size of an oven tray, or a stew or low GI vegetable ensemble that can go with protein meals, and put it in the fridge. This way you have the food sitting there ready to go and you can grab something for lunch, and when you come home in the evening you can heat something up for dinner. Normally with me lunch is the main meal, so at my clinic I have a barbecue outside that I throw something on to quickly cook while I heat up some vegies or make a fresh salad to go with it. In the evening I will eat whatever is in the fridge. The fresh pasta is also a good standby, because it only takes a few minutes to cook. You can also get the meals home-delivered.

3. **Eat more of the protein meals in the first few weeks.** When you eat more of the protein meals to start off with you get a more dramatic result. You will see the kilos dropping off. The reason is your body has become so used to getting all the free energy it wants from the high GI carbs it becomes lazy. When this suddenly disappears, the body starts furiously burning up the fat to compensate for the lack of glucose, but after a few weeks it starts to settle down and burns the fat more efficiently, usually around 500g–1kg (1 to 2 pounds) a week on average. One has to take advantage of this and hit the body at full speed. So

more protein meals for the first few weeks. That means a few protein breakfasts during the week, bacon and eggs or perhaps an omelette, and protein lunches and dinners the rest of the time. Of course include plenty of the low GI vegetables with this, you need your fibre, but what you should discover is that after a couple of weeks of this you should see quite an improvement with your weight.

This is also a useful technique if you find that you have hit a 'plateau' for a while. Eating more protein meals can get you started again, but we will discuss this in more detail later on.

What can I expect?

I have made a list of the main things you could expect to anticipate when doing everything right.

1. **Very pleasing weight loss:** As I have said before, on average the weight usually comes off between 500g–1kg (1–2 pounds) per week. With some people it can be more, others it can be less – one way or another you should be very pleased with how it comes off. This aspect usually outweighs the concerns about having to make certain changes to your eating pattern.

2. **Sugar withdrawals:** In the first few days, after dropping the sugar and high GI carbs from the diet, a person can experience withdrawals. Usually this is nothing more than

feeling the desire for 'something sweet' and it usually passes after a day or three but for some this is not always the case. The higher the person's exposure to sugars and high GI carbs over the course of a lifetime, the bigger the withdrawals will be. For those people who have made 'a career' out of eating high GI carbs, you can expect confusion, headaches, lethargy, sugar craving and depression. The good news is these symptoms are only transient and normally take no longer than a week to pass. Once it's over, it's over and you feel like a new person. The high GI carbs are like a drug to the body and the bigger the withdrawals the more you were hooked! Essentially this phase is a good learning experience.

3. **Lack of food craving:** Another pleasing experience that many people comment on is the fact that a lot of foods that you could not live without lose their attraction. This can come as quite a surprise, especially to people whose whole lives revolved around certain foods. No longer being a slave to food makes you free at last, and this can also be highly motivating for people.

4. **Eating more if you like, but eventually eating less:** Another thing that you may find is although you can eat the protein meals as much as you like and the carb meals in moderation, you may find that eventually, over time, the amount you eat starts to become more conservative because you feel full sooner. There are a few theories about why it happens but for the time being this is just something that you will need to experience yourself.

5. **Being able to buy new clothes:** Who hasn't enjoyed some 'retail therapy' from time to time. But when one is overweight, buying new clothes can be a pain. On one hand you have to pay good money for some items and on the other they don't always make you look that much better. I can clearly remember the trouble I had BGI (before the GI) when buying clothes. I used to actually try to avoid it and ended up wearing the same old clothes. I spent my twenties being taut, trim and athletic, only to put on weight the further I got into my thirties. I think a lot of people can relate to this. How often have I heard people say 'I used to be able to eat anything I liked'. Many people go out looking for clothes after they have dropped the weight, and discover they are a few sizes smaller. It is extremely pleasing. Even getting something out of the wardrobe that once fitted, to find that you once again can wear it, gives you quite a thrill. Some people have told me that just being able to go into a store and buy something off the rack is fantastic, as often their size had not even been stocked. So be prepared to do a little spending on some new outfits.

6. **People's comments:** Just remember this: when you are overweight, people will not comment. Only people very, very close to you will say anything. Often, because no one says anything, a person gets the impression that no one seems to notices the extra kilograms. The acid test is when you lose the weight. People will start to comment. It usually starts with 'Gee, you're looking well' but continues on to people saying 'My god have you lost weight'? And so on.

173

From my experience I have met many people when they were overweight only to meet them again after they have lost the weight and not recognise them. This happens. Something else happens when they transform themselves. What immediately happens is the opposite sex finds them very attractive, and the next thing you know they are having trouble with all the attention they are getting. Amazing as this may seem many people have never been in a situation where they are really attractive to the opposite sex, and it can be anxious for some (others take to it like a duck to water). Fortunately for those who need a little coaching, I have a lecture on what to look for in a partner which goes part of the way to stabilising the situation.

7. **Spending more money on fresh food:** Quite simply, you will have discovered that just about every off-the-shelf food contains sugar or some other starch as an ingredient. The number of canned/packaged foods that are low GI in supermarkets you can count on one hand. So as a result you are buying fresh produce each week. It may add to the food bill because you're not padding out your shopping with junk, but the upside is your health. Always remember, 'maintenance is cheaper than repair'. Look after your weight and you probably won't get a problem with your health.

8. **Increased energy and wellbeing:** A frequent observation by many people is the feeling of wellbeing. This is often because they are not suffering the peaks and troughs in their blood sugar levels, which goes a long way towards

improving their energy levels. The other thing is you are not experiencing the effect that high GI carbs have on your appetite and, as a result, not overeating. Not having to worry about food and your weight also adds to peace of mind.

9. **Not bloated after a meal:** Another aspect to avoiding the high GI foods is there is a distinct lack of bloating and distension in the stomach. The reason for this is the surplus glucose found in the high GI carbs causes a fermentation to occur with the bacteria in the gut. This in turn leads to gas building up in the intestines and we all know what that leads to . . . (pardon me, did someone step on a duck!?!) Without the glucose this doesn't occur and one finds that bloating is completely absent even after you have had a big meal.

10. **Getting constipated in the first week or so:** This only happens to a few people but if it's you, then what's going on is you are probably eating more protein. Meat generally is harder to digest and for some people that can make them sluggish. The other reason is the afore-mentioned lack of bloating is gone and the gas which used to pressurise the gut is also gone. This gas acts in the same way champagne tries to push the cork out of the bottle – it helps push things through the intestines. This is also a transient phase, which passes usually after the first week. The cure for this is to simply add more fibre to your breakfast, to help things along. Your body's own peristaltic action strengthens over time and normality returns.

11. **Get disappointed when you eat high GI carbs:** Because you make the effort to avoid the high GI carbs, there's a part of your mind that thinks you're missing out on something or being denied. So for one reason or another you'll find an excuse to eat something you shouldn't. Be prepared for disappointment. Sure it will taste good – that's your brain's chemistry trying to tell you that if you had any second thoughts about not eating it, don't bother. It's a high energy food source, but you will be surprised to discover that it wasn't as good as you were expecting.

    More acutely, shortly afterwards you may find that you are starting to feel like rubbish. Your blood sugar levels are starting to crash, and it's around now that your body seems to say 'What are you doing, everything was going along fine and now you've had to go and spoil it'. It's a good learning experience for some people and I have to admit for the first few years, I still got a buzz out of eating the occasional thing I knew probably wasn't doing me any favours, but as time went by to my surprise even those occasions started to lose their attraction. Many of my patients have told me of similar experiences – don't be surprised when it happens to you.

12. **Not worrying about your weight:** As I have explained already it's not just about weight, but there are many problems that flow on from being overweight. Heart disease, diabetes and so on. These should all be in the past for you once you understand about using the GI. Once you have got the weight down and been cruising

along just maintaining your weight and having the occasional night out only to discover you have inadvertently gained a few extra kilos, just simply do things 'by the book' again and it will come off just as easily as before.

So by now you should be starting to follow the meal planner. Just remember that it is intended as a guide as to how to structure your eating. You can change things around to suit your individual tastes. We have a recipe book called *GI Feel Good: Meals Made Easy* if you need more suggestions and you can get new recipes each week from the website. Like I said earlier you can also get the food delivered to your home depending on which city you live in.

CHAPTER 3

Being happy with your choices

You may be surprised as to how many things are related to blood sugar levels and the wonders of insulin. By controlling that one little thing gives you a handle on a variety of different problems. Here are a few of them.

Caution: diatribe ahead.

Obesity and diabetes

Any medical professional knows that obesity and diabetes go hand-in-hand. In countries where the number of overweight people is increasing, diabetes is also on the increase. Diabetes is becoming one of the largest health problems currently faced by the West. Of course the leader is the US but Australia is coming second! There is something seriously wrong.

The number of obese Australian adults has climbed dramatically over the past decade and will continue to soar in coming years. While 2.4 million adults already fall into the obese category, this figure will rise 12.5 per cent by 2010. Researchers have found that the proportion of obese Australians has increased by almost 80 per cent over the past 13 years.

At least 16 per cent of men and 17 per cent of women aged 18 and older are now obese, with a further 42 per cent of men and 25 per cent of women classified as overweight. Australia's highest levels of obesity are among people aged 35 to 69. With an ageing populating, an extra 300,000 people would be obese by 2010 – with a further 600,000 falling into the same category by 2020.

Australia still has an adult-obesity rate (16 per cent) lower than that in the US (21 per cent), but the rate of obesity is increasing at similar rates in both countries.

The proportion of obese and overweight Australians is already the same as the American figure in 1995.

The image of sun-bronzed Aussies stomping their way across a golden beach is giving way to the couch potatoes sprawled in front of TV, surrounded by empty drink cans and pizza boxes.

Whether we want to blame lack of exercise or the proliferation of fast food companies, we have to face it, the problem is a very real one and most disturbingly it is now affecting our most precious assets. The young.

Childhood obesity has had a three-fold increase since 1985 with one in five children being overweight and almost one in ten children obese. That means about 30% of children are overweight or obese, an alarming statistic. Not only is diabetes waiting in the wings, children as young as seven and eight are showing signs of arteriosclerosis, an adult heart disease found in people three to five times their age.

No amount of hand-wringing is going to solve the problem. People need to know what to do with their diets and in particular understand how to use the GI. I will discuss later what to do about overweight kiddies using the GI but for now I would just like to focus on diabetes.

People will develop diabetes for two main reason. First there are those who have a defect with the pancreas and it has problems functioning properly. This usually shows up early on in life and is the less common form of the illness. There can be a number of factors that can lead to this. It can be genetic, viral, autoimmune or related to diet. This is called type I diabetes and often occurs early during childhood. The other type is more common and this is where the pancreas starts to have problems with keeping up with the demand for insulin and starts to pack it in. This can happen later in life, hence the term 'mature onset' or type II diabetes. There are also hereditary factors with this but the biggest risk factor is obesity. In this situation the person can take medication to keep their blood sugar levels under control but may have to start taking medication to replace the insulin the pancreas would otherwise produce, hence the terms 'insulin dependent' and 'non-insulin dependent' diabetics.

Unfortunately, if it was simply a matter of replacing the missing insulin then that would be the end of it. However there are further and even more severe problems associated with long-term diabetes, which include cardiovascular illness, circulation problems, eye problems, cognitive problems and, possibly most disturbing, the loss of feet and legs. Naturally the one stand-out treatment for preventing diabetes is losing the weight and keeping your blood sugar levels under control by diet.

Once a person has developed insulin dependent diabetes, a low GI diet is not going to make them better, however every so often I get the occasional letter from non-insulin dependent diabetics who have read the book and discovered that by following my advice, they have reportedly kept their blood sugar levels under control for many months at a time. This is usually achieved with little or no medication at all. Naturally I am not suggesting people not take their medication, but what they are telling me is that there is no need to use their blood sugar lowering medication because their BSLs are not elevated by their food. This, in my opinion, would have a very positive effect on reducing deterioration over time and hopefully prevent the person from developing the insulin dependent version of the illness.

One would expect that every diabetic organisation in the country would be espousing a low GI diet; unfortunately this has not been the case. Why? I have my own theories but suffice to say it's not on the immediate agenda. A low GI diet takes the strain off the pancreas having to keep up with the daily production of insulin, while on a conventional diet it's struggling to keep up with the demand. Besides this the other health benefits of weight loss and lowering of cholesterol, two other factors associated with diabetes, are also addressed. Keeping our blood sugar levels under control is the obvious answer to preventing diabetes and last time I checked, 'an ounce of prevention is worth a pound of cure'. But remember this, when it comes to the big end of town, there's money in treatment and no money in cure. Understanding the GI and having the ability to prevent a variety of problems has only cost you a little of your time and the price of this book. A small investment that can last a lifetime.

Hypoglycemia

You may have heard about hypoglycemia and thought it one of those 'fad' types of problems. Well, it's real enough and you would have probably experienced it every time you have a lunch with the high GI carbs. Hypoglycemia is what happens when your blood sugar level falls below the normal amount. The type of symptoms that can occur include: fatigue, mental confusion, mild depression and withdrawal, irritability, lack of concentration and digestive disturbances. Having read this far, you may already have some insight into why hypoglycemia has suddenly become such a problem over the past few years. Western medicine still struggles to recognise that hypo-glycemia actually exists outside of insulin dependent diabetics and, as I alluded to earlier, it's the reason you feel tired in the afternoon a few hours after lunch.

Some people hardly notice the change in their blood sugar levels but for others, usually those who's energy levels are already pretty low already, it can really hit them, and quite often it is they who will eventually try to find some professional help.

Naturally, if the person turns up at my office, I am always keen to see what difference taking all the high GI carb out of the diet has. This is often the most direct route to eliminating the symptoms. Building up the energy levels is another matter. Quite often the person tells me the advice from the doctor was to eat barley sugar to get their blood sugar levels back up again. It makes sense but what the doctor is forgetting is that the elevated blood sugar levels caused the condition in the first place.

What occurs is the high GI carbohydrates raise the blood sugar level past the point where insulin is released. What then happens is the pancreas, after years of having to pump out insulin to combat the blood sugar level, eventually gets run down and starts to overcompensate. Instead of releasing the exact amount of insulin needed to lower the blood sugar levels, the pancreas develops a knee-jerk reaction to high GI carbohydrates. When the blood sugar levels go shooting up, the pancreas reacts by releasing too much insulin into the bloodstream. What typically occurs is the excess insulin drives the blood sugar levels way down. By metabolising and getting rid of the glucose, a person can go from having too much glucose in the blood, to not enough.

The actual mechanics are more like this: what initially happens after you eat high GI carbs is for the first half-hour the blood sugar level starts to rise. Insulin is then released, and over the next half hour the insulin metabolises the excess blood sugar, and it begins to drive the glucose down to its normal limit. But because the pancreas has overcompensated, there is an excess of insulin excreted. This excess continues to convert the glucose in the blood, lowering the blood sugar level even further. As a result, you begin to experience hypoglycemia.

This will continue for the next two hours. During this time the first thing that you will notice is tiredness as you start nodding off at your desk (that is if you are behind a desk and not the wheel of a car!). You can also experience a kind of 'brain fog' and find it difficult to concentrate. There is another over-riding quality to this hypoglycemic phase. During the next two hours you will also have cravings for more high GI carbs to get your blood sugar levels back up again. This is perfectly natural.

Your body at this time does not have enough glucose in the bloodstream, and as a result it is telling you to eat something that will produce more glucose. The interesting part is you will tend to overlook things that have a moderate GI as the body is in a sort of 'crisis situation', and will steer you towards the high GI carb every time.

> Studies have shown that the inclusion of bad carbs in a person's diet causes a tendency to eat 20% more food than normal.

Here we have the basis of sugar craving and sugar addiction. Because you are now craving more sugar, it is very likely that you will eat another high GI carbohydrate, pushing up the blood sugar level, and starting the whole process again. Three hours or so after eating the initial high GI carbohydrates, you once again start scrounging around for something else.

The pancreas responds in the same way again and on and on we go. That is why you can still feel hungry a few hours after a meal and crave sweet food. By now you are probably realising that it is a three-hour roller coaster going up and down three times a day, every day. If we have to overcompensate with our eating, then inevitably gaining weight is going to be a problem. This is a vicious cycle that I feel is at the heart of a lot of eating problems. A low GI diet eliminates this.

Metabolic Syndrome – Syndrome X and IRS

This is something else you may stumble upon and I should point out that it is an emerging study – I am sure there will be more information coming to light at the time of publishing this book. Metabolic Syndrome or Syndrome X was first noticed in 1988. It is a collection of symptoms that came to be first known as Syndrome X, and then was referred to as Metabolic Syndrome. The WHO already has an MS (multiple sclerosis) and didn't like the sound of SX – they want it to be referred to as Insulin Resistance Syndrome (IRS), but here in Australia we call it Metabolic Syndrome or Syndrome X.

Basically, this is a condition where the person has abnormally high BSLs and insulin in the blood all the time. The problem is that the cells are not accepting the sugar. This is commonly seen in obese or overweight people who also present with high cholesterol and triglycerides levels and hypertension (high blood pressure). What happens is when the person is pumping out lots of insulin, usually because of eating high GI carbs all the time, the body gets

186

tired of being bombarded with the glucose and the insulin and starts to resist it. The glucose and insulin just float around in the blood instead of being absorbed and you are left with abnormally high insulin and blood sugar levels all the time. So how does this apply to the GI if you have this condition? In the short term, it means the difference between a person who can eat plenty of moderate carbs and still have the weight come off and a person who finds the weight comes off slowly or not at all.

Occasionally on our website forum, we will have a person who eats lots of moderate carbs and seems to be able to bend the rules and not have it affect them. This sort of person probably does not have this condition. However occasionally there's a person who does everything right, but may be leaning a little more towards the moderate carbs. In some cases this sort of person can plateau or find their weight loss hang or slow for no obvious reason. This is usually because the person is affected by metabolic syndrome and the result is they get a slightly higher rise in the BSLs than normal. What this means in real terms is that, if the safety margin for moderate carbs is a GI of 50 or below, this person may find that their personal safety margin may be 40 or below.

In practice that's the reason behind 'being moderate with the moderate carbs', just in case a person goes overboard and starts eating tonnes of moderate carbs to compensate for the lack of sugar in their diet and brings themselves undone. If the person has Metabolic Syndrome then they are getting more 'bang for your buck' when they eat moderate carbs. They have to take it easy with the moderate carbs and eat more of the low GI or excellent carbs.

What researchers believe is IRS is a precursor to type II diabetes, although observations show that people can have this condition for several years without going on to develop diabetes. Researchers believe that weight gain, hereditary factors, sedentary lifestyles, overeating and age may also be related. Again, it's not one of these problems that you wake up and discover you have one morning, it comes on slowly over time. If you have been persistently overweight for a number of years you may find that you could be affected by this condition. The good news is a low GI diet gradually fixes the condition over time as well, so in the meantime just don't go overboard on the moderate carbs.

The West's consumption of sugar

The World Health Organization (WHO) met in 2004 for its 57th annual assembly to tackle what's regarded as the greatest crisis in public health today – obesity. But already there are claims that industry lobby groups are trying to undermine the WHO's proposed strategy that would see governments around the world backing healthier diets and more exercise.

The scientific debate has become so heated that the fight to defend the sugar industry has been compared by some to the battle over tobacco. The tactics used by the industry lobby groups are the same as Big Tobacco. It's simple, just keep attacking the scientific evidence – 'there's no proof smoking causes lung cancer', for example.

But there's a lot at stake, with WHO figures estimating there are more than one billion overweight adults worldwide – at least three hundred million of them obese. That's adults and doesn't include children.

The reason why there is so much excitement in the sugar industry is because it was one of the culprits singled out by the WHO and because of this the Australian government has come under pressure to implement some of the recommendations. Strangely enough the US isn't having a bar of the recommendations and Australia is towing the US line. Ho hum . . .

We can no longer go down the road of simply telling everybody it's a good idea to have a balanced diet because in fact we have to have strategic developments by governments.

Governments, including Australia's, were among the critics of the first global attempt to battle obesity by rallying nations under the World Health Organization banner.

When the WHO released its wide-ranging draft Global Strategy on Diet, Physical Activity and Health it came under fire from countries including the US and Australia, as well as the sugar industry and big food companies.

PROFESSOR PHILIP JAMES, INTERNATIONAL OBESITY TASK FORCE

The title of our first book was *Sugar Science* and interestingly enough, we sold hundreds of copies to Bundaberg, Australia's sugar capital in Queensland. The simple fact is sugar is in just about everything we get off the shelf. People have even discovered sugar as an ingredient of mineral water. When you start looking you will be as amazed as I was as to how much food contains sugar. In fact there are only two items that we buy from the supermarket that do not contain sugar: they are a can of tinned mushrooms and an imported Italian tomato paste. Think about it for a moment next time you go to the supermarket. Look at the rows upon rows of products that contain sugar and think about the size of the industry needed to supply that one commodity on such a large-scale to every food shop and supermarket in the country, and also to every country in the world. It's really mind-boggling. Suffice to say, the battle hasn't even started yet.

The story as to how sugar has become such a huge commodity is worthy of a book all on its own. (A really great documentary on the subject is called 'The Politics of Food'. See if you can find it.)

It is estimated that Westerners' consumption of sugar has risen from 2.5 kg (5 pounds) a year in the 1800s to a staggering 90 kg (180 pounds) a year in 1990. In a study here in Australia, *Choice* magazine put together a survey of the top ten items in peoples' shopping trolleys. What do you expect they found? Milk, bread, veggies? *Choice* reported that the top four items were in fact cola drinks! What would you expect that to be doing to one's health?

The WHO is also targeting fat as another culprit, and lack of exercise, and what we are seeing from them is a clearer message than the original ineffectual version of 'we should all be eating a balanced diet', which is meaningless to most overweight people. What people need is a strategy. In my opinion the GI is the pinnacle of our understanding and in the next 20 to 30 years you will see the GI on everything. Time will be the judge.

Cholesterol and high insulin levels

Cholesterol is something that we hear a lot about, but it can be a little confusing to really understand. High cholesterol is linked to the increased risk of heart attack. So lowering cholesterol has been a catch cry for more than 15 years, but how do we actually do it? Well you can take medication. Pfizer, the pharmaceutical giant, sells a lipid-lowering anti-cholesterol drug called Lipitor. The company's reported sales of the drug, the world's largest-selling pharmaceutical, rose 19 per cent in the first quarter of 2004 to $2.497 billion. On the other hand you can try to not eat fats and things that contain cholesterol, which is what your GP will tell you, but it has also been noted that the persistent presence of a high insulin level in the blood also increases the level of cholesterol and triglycerides. These two factors have been held mostly responsible for blocked arteries and heart disease.

Over the years I have recommended that patients suffering from high cholesterol levels follow my advice, and avoid the high GI carbohydrates to keep their insulin level under control. Remember that fats, including cholesterol, cannot be stored without insulin. In every case upon re-examination by their regular doctor, patients have reported a fall in their cholesterol level, sometimes quite dramatically. One doctor even described it as 'a miracle'.

When you have your cholesterol checked there are three readings. One for the good cholesterol or HDL (high density lipoprotein), one the bad cholesterol LDL (low density lipoprotein) and another for the triglycerides. Make sure you understand that it is the LDL reading that matters. The number the doctor gives you is the sum of the two.

At the beginning of this year I read a delightful story about an 88-year-old man who lived in an old people's home. Apparently the gentleman suffered from dementia and had an 'egg' fixation. As a result he ate up to 26 eggs a day for a total of 15 years. The local doctor, upon hearing about this gentleman's condition, couldn't contain his excitement and rushed off to take a blood sample, expecting his cholesterol levels to be through the roof. To the doctor's utter amazement the results indicated that his cholesterol levels were normal. Unfortunately the doctor was unable to understand why this was and went on to write a report about this extraordinary man and the cholesterol anomaly, which is how I ended up reading about it. After understanding this much about the GI, can you possibly think why his cholesterol levels were normal? Firstly eggs are protein, and do not contain carbohydrate, so it didn't matter how much the man ate, they had no effect on his blood sugar levels, so his body was unable to retain the cholesterol which is found in the yolk of the egg. Of course the gentleman seemed to only eat eggs – if he was eating toast with his eggs, as just about everyone else does, his cholesterol would be off the scale.

So you are probably wondering what happens to the fat and cholesterol while on a low GI diet. We had always said that the body doesn't absorb it, because we knew from experience people ate fat in their diets and lost weight *and* their cholesterol levels were fine. However it has only been in the last few years that we have found out more about it. But first let's learn about the way fats are dealt within the body.

Fats are absorbed in the first part of the digestive tract after they leave the stomach. The liver releases bile, which adds itself to the fats to make an emulsion and causes the fats to go into globules or molecules to be absorbed. At the same time the pancreas releases 'juices', which allows the fats to be transported into the blood.

The fats come in two varieties; High Density Lipoproteins (HDLs) and Low Density Lipoproteins (LDLs). These are more commonly referred to as 'good fats' and 'bad fats'. Now assuming that the person has no idea about the GI and has been eating bad carbs with their fats, when the two go into the bloodstream the insulin acts upon them causing them to shrink. The HDL, being so dense, hardly shrinks and spends the next few hours going around and rubbing away at the artery walls, cleaning them much like detergent, before being reabsorbed by the liver and passing back out in the bile and carried away with the waste. What's 'good' about them is they collect and carry away plaque that causes blood clots that lead to heart disease and they are often referred to as plaque scavengers.

The LDLs, or bad fats, also float around in the blood, but what happens is the insulin comes along and shrinks them also. The LDLs are not as dense and the insulin succeeds in making them small enough to be absorbed by the body. Why they are 'bad' is because they pass through the artery walls and leave deposits of cholesterol behind, which in turn causes bulges in the artery walls. These bulges act like speed humps which the red blood cells 'bump' as they whiz around in the blood. These bumps make bruises in the artery walls, which in turn lead to the body putting little tiles or 'plaque' over the bruises to protect the artery from further damage. Unfortunately these plaque patches can break off unexpectedly and travel through the blood until it hits a bottleneck where it causes a blood clot. If it's an artery to the heart you have a massive heart attack. If it's the brain you have a stroke and may survive with partial paralysis down one side.

What happens when you include fats in the diet *and* keep your BSLs under control is very, very interesting and the subject of research in the US.

The fats still get the same treatment by the bile and the pancreatic juices as before, but when they arrive in the bloodstream there's no insulin to meet them. As a result the two molecules stay the same size. The LDLs or, so-called bad fats, act in the same way as the HDLs, or so-called good fats. They both go on their merry way scouring the arteries and cleaning away the plaque, before passing back out of the body via the liver. This normally happens 4–5 hours later. So believe it or not the fat in the diet, besides not doing any harm, is actually help-ing prevent heart disease. A very significant and satisfying outcome.

Anaerobic bacteria and sugar

In the digestive tract there is a combination of bacteria that is referred to as the body's normal intestinal flora. The body needs this to aid in the digestion of food. These bacteria fall into two types: one that prefers oxygen and the other that prefers sugar. Both aerobic and anaerobic bacteria use oxygen to burn sugar, but because the anaerobic bacteria doesn't use very much oxygen, it requires about four times more sugar to survive. Anaerobic bacteria, although a necessary part of the intestinal flora, are not required in great abundance. The aerobic bacteria are however, and they keep the presence of the anaerobic bacteria in check. When there is too much glucose from high

GI carbs passing through the digestive tract, then the anaerobic bacteria have a very good opportunity to thrive. The presence of an overabundance of anaerobic bacteria causes digestive disturbances.

Instead of aiding in the breakdown of foods like aerobic bacteria do, anaerobic bacteria tend to cause more of a fermentation to occur. You will probably notice that when you eat sugars and bad carbohydrates, it is very common to experience bloating afterwards. This is normally the result of the anaerobic bacteria causing the food to ferment because of the presence of excess sugar. Conversely, bloating can be a sure sign that you have eaten the wrong kinds of carbs. Further complications can ensue if this situation is left unchecked. The bloating causes the abdomen to distend and stretch the surrounding adipose tissue, making it more accessible for fat to accumulate. This is why people develop a beer gut, for example. The combination of the carbohydrate and yeast from the beer causes both distension and weight gain simultaneously. Yeast is something that also thrives on sugar.

Back in the 80s and 90s naturopaths were telling people they suffered from candida. It is a type of yeast that can cause a number of problems when it gets out of hand. Unfortunately the list of ailments was quite extensive. It was blamed for anything from bad breath to psychosis. The funny thing about this is that candida occurs naturally in the body so it is always possible to find it. That didn't seem to matter very much because naturopaths were making a fortune from telling people that they had it. Nowadays, the big candida scare has come and gone and telling everybody that they are suffering from candida is a thing of the past. Please don't misunderstand me, candida is a genuine problem, but it is still a symptom rather than a disease. I think the latest manifestation of the problem is now irritable bowel syndrome (IBS), again the description for a collection of symptoms.

Finding out why the person has the problem in the first place, rather than just treating the symptoms, is the very cornerstone of Traditional Chinese Medicine (TCM). Discovering the cause provides you with the answer.

Besides avoiding yeast, the problems of candida are best avoided by not filling yourself with high GI carbs and sugar. When a person presents with these types of symptoms, the first thing that I do is remove all the bad carbohydrates from their diet. I have attended patients with severe digestive problems that even specialists could not help, only to have a complete reversal of their symptoms after taking out the bad carbs. I have always taken the approach of removing the bad carbs first, because if nothing happens then I know that it's not the sugar causing the symptoms – we can then start narrowing down the field of other possibilities. The Chinese approach is to look at the obvious first and if that's not it *then* start eliminating. Western Medicine, conversely, starts at the opposite end by eliminating everything and then reintroducing things one by one.

Another way that the intestinal flora can become out of balance is for a person to take antibiotics. Antibiotics often kill off both types of bacteria and once the course is finished, the body has to re-establish the bacterial community to function properly. Of course, if there is a lot of bad carbohydrate passing through the digestive tract, then the anaerobic bacteria and yeast get a headstart and can dominate.

This is why problems like diarrhoea commonly ensue after taking antibiotics, and why it is recommended that you have acidophilus once the antibiotics are finished. Acidophilus can reflorinate the gut with the good bacteria and circumvent any problems. You can find it in yoghurt, but there are also tablets and drinks that are specifically designed to deliver the bacteria to the intestines, and it should only be a one-off treatment. Whichever product you choose, just be sure that it doesn't contain sugar. Even though sugar exacerbates the problem, some manufacturers still add sugar to their product so people will like it. What the . . .?

Polycystic Ovarian Syndrome (PCOS)

PCOS is a major cause of infertility and it is something that I see patients for quite regularly. Ultrasound routinely reveals that up to 20 per cent of women in the reproductive age range have polycystic ovaries. Of that number about half as many or approximately six to ten per cent will be effected by the condition, which is characterised by irregular or absent periods and elevated hormone levels (in particular testosterone and androstenedione). Patients with this syndrome may complain of abnormal bleeding, infertility, obesity, excess hair growth, hair loss and acne. In addition to the clinical and hormonal changes associated with this, ultrasounds also show enlarged ovaries with an increased number of small (six to ten mm) follicles around the periphery of the ovary, hence the name poly (many) cystic (cysts or pimples) around the ovaries.

Some people can have a genetic reason for developing this condition. They may have both male and female relatives with adult-onset diabetes, obesity, elevated blood triglycerides, high blood pressure and female relatives with infertility, hormonal and menstrual problems. Many thousands of years ago the Chinese also realised that women had this problem, but interestingly they came to the conclusion that the problem was caused by 'sweet things', or in other words, sugar and high GI foods.

I read some years ago that in the US doctors found that a low carb diet is essential for treating PCOS. I was quite pleased because I had been putting women on a low carb diet for several years already, and had developed quite a reputation for helping women become pregnant (I don't know why audiences think that is so hilarious . . .?). I had always known through my training in TCM that it was related to the blood sugar levels and I had most of my success by modifying the patient's diet and also using traditional herbal medicine to boost the woman's fertility.

Western medicine has got as far as understanding the connection between PCOS and insulin. What has been decided is that the person has had abnormally high insulin levels in the blood for many years. This gave rise to another discovery and a new syndrome called 'insulin resistant syndrome' or syndrome X, as previously discussed. Suffice to say the person has a persistently high insulin level and this in turn affects the ovaries. Instead of the ovary producing an egg each month and having it slide down the fallopian tube to the womb, the egg instead hangs around the ovaries and becomes a cyst, like a pimple. Each month the ovary produces another egg and each month another little pimple appears. When the nurse comes along with the ultrasound, she sees all these little 'pimples' around the ovary.

Another interesting aspect is the connection between being overweight and PCOS. The excess body fat actually starts to convert the hormone estrogen into testosterone, hence the onset of facial hair and acne that's also seen with the condition. Naturally having your estrogen changed into testosterone is not going to do much for a woman's fertility. Besides being one of the main reasons for not becoming pregnant, PCOS causes other problems.

A syndrome is a collection of symptoms or problems, all grouped under the one heading, meaning we know that they all have something to do with each other, although we may not always know how or why. Other things that can be related to PCOS are irregular periods, and even no periods, or breakthrough bleeding and spotting. In Australia the doctor routinely turns to an insulin-lowering drug called 'Metformin', which can sometimes alleviate some of the symptoms. As with all medication it carries a risk of side effects. Naturally keeping your blood sugar levels under control by following a low GI diet would be the obvious solution. It's the approach I have taken and quite often the lady falls pregnant as the cysts go away, skin clears up and so on. The facial hair is a little more tricky and is usually an indicator that the problem has been around for many years already and has become a chronic problem. In this situation I usually suspect that the person may be also developing a fibroid, and may need to see a gynaecologist about having it removed, although I have had patients with fibroids follow the book only to find after a few months the fibroids shrinking and eventually disappearing.

Interestingly, the Chinese recognised that women developed fibroids a century ago and again also believed that it was related to sugar.

Another problem with PCOS is that women with the condition who do conceive can have a higher risk of miscarriage. Although the research has shown a correlation between women with PCOS and miscarriages, there may be other hereditary factors also. Quite often once a doctor had made the diagnosis of PCOS the patient will think it is a condition that they have for life. I try to encourage people to think of it as a transient condition that can eventually go away. Why? Because from experience, in a lot of cases the cysts eventually do go away. PCOS isn't something that just happens all of a sudden, it's a chronic condition that develops over many years. It is not unusual for a patient who has maintained a good eating regime, as per the GI, to find that eventually the PCOS has gone.

Less insulin keeps you younger

Massachusetts General Hospital in Boston made a remarkable discovery about a particular gene that can slow the cellular ageing process in human beings. Guess what? The gene is switched on and off by insulin. Cells obtain energy by combining glucose with oxygen, a process called metabolic oxidation, which inevitably creates highly reactive atoms called free radicals. Free radicals can damage DNA and disrupt healthy cells. When cells become damaged, the body quickly replaces them. Free radical damage is one of the things that causes premature ageing. One only needs to look at smokers to see the premature ageing that is a result of free radical damage. The chemical in cigarette smoke produces an enormous number of free radicals and as we all know free radicals damage DNA and can lead to diseases like cancer.

Experiments with mice on low carbohydrate diets have demonstrated that when insulin is not being released, this newly-discovered gene switches on and causes the cells in the body to begin to burn glucose at a highly efficient rate. There is a correlation to human counterparts. Many patients have also reported a remarkable lift in their energy levels accompanied with the weight loss (as well as a curious desire for cheese . . . coincidence?).

Because the cells are now operating more efficiently, there is less oxidation occurring, and as a result, less damaging free radicals are being formed. Not only did the mice have more energy, they also lived longer, up to 40 per cent longer than their litter mates on an unrestricted diet. It has been observed that people who live for an extraordinarily long time and typically survive on a low GI diet are often thin. They avoid the peaks in their blood sugar level, unlike people on an unrestricted diet. Credible evidence from research on native peoples, like the herdsmen of Pakistan's Hunza valley and the Indians of Mexico's Sierra Madre mountains, who live on simple and Spartan diets shows that they do live longer and that a few can reach a remarkable age.

More recent research has also shown that if mice are allowed to eat between 20–30 per cent less food, then their life expectancy extends dramatically. People on a long-term low GI diet eat about 20 per cent less than average. Scientists have concluded that the life expectancy on such a diet could go as high as 130 years. Now if you are anything like me and the thought of wandering around at the ripe old age of 130 years doesn't exactly thrill you, then you should be thinking about it as a means to age more slowly and keep your youthful looks much longer.

Being able to stay the same weight forever

After I had become very familiar with the GI and lost the extra weight, it soon became apparent that the problem of putting on weight as I grew older had also gone. If you haven't realised already, the GI is one of the fundamental reasons why you gain, lose or maintain your weight and therefore the ability to control your weight is within your control now that you know how to use the GI.

I have been using this knowledge now for more than a decade and I am always pleased at how well it works so many years down the track. Prior to all this I reconciled myself to the fact that as one grew older, we generally gather weight. The average person gains roughly half a kilogram each year once past the age of 30, which means by the age of 40 you will be five kilos (10 pounds) heavier, 10 kilos (20 pounds) by the age of 50 and so on and so on.

Being in some ways like my dad, I became aware that I might end up taking after him when I got older, a bit on the heavy side, stocky and barrel-chested. Unfortunately for dad, he died way too young, at age 64 from heart attack. Don't worry; I was only 12 and too young to have helped him with his eating habits. If only I had known then what I know now, things may have been different.

An inevitable consequence of understanding how to use the GI is that you should never need to worry about your weight as long as you use the principles of the GI. Many of my patients, like myself, have turned their lives around forever. This above all things is one of the most satisfying for me. Once you have achieved your goals and mastered this knowledge, for

202

the rest of your life you carry a powerful tool that can be used again and again as the need arises. The section on maintaining your health goes into more practical detail on this subject and is useful for the long-term.

Binge eating

As the name implies, binge eating is when the people can't stop overeating. The body actually has mechanisms to tell you to stop but we learn to override these, usually when we are young. Having to finish everything on the plate before leaving the table is a good example.

Overeating can give people a high and allow them to compensate for other things missing in their life. One of my patients even told me that they found eating was like having sexual relations! Don't get me wrong, I enjoy eating but I draw the line at installing a mirror over the kitchen table.

When the person focuses completely on eating and ignores the tell-tale signals that they are full, they end up eating too much. One of the more common patterns I see is when the person doesn't eat very much during the day, avoids eating breakfast, but goes home at night and binge eats. This is not very healthy. Of course when they get up in the morning, as is always the case after having a big meal the night before, they don't feel like eating and the cycle repeats itself again.

I often see young people who starve themselves, sometimes for a day or so in an effort to lose weight, before giving in to the hunger and bingeing again. Of course this just precipitates the process again. This causes enormous problems for the digestion as well as the person's self-image and self-esteem.

Binge eating can often be a form of compensatory behaviour for other things, however it can also have something to do with the amount of insulin being produced.

When we eat something that gives us a big rise in blood sugar levels and a surplus of insulin, the excess insulin actually binds to receptors in the brain to produce sugar cravings, and this is the signal for us to overeat again. Another crazy thing the body does is to reward us for eating high energy food. It's one of those ancient survival mechanism that I spoke about earlier. That's why we go 'mmm yummy' when we eat things that maybe we shouldn't. Is it really yummy or is it because our brains tell us that it is yummy? The brain actually makes us 'think' it's yummy by releasing chemicals to make us want to eat it, just in case we were having second thoughts. You see, our body wants the food more than we do and it will override us if it can. The good news is that when we stop presenting the high energy food to it, it stops and as a result people lose their food cravings. After a little while you will wonder why you ever ate the things you did. What I find ironic is that in spite of *our* ignorance, our bodies have known about GI for a very long time. When you look at the types of food that most people prefer, it is no coincidence that it's almost always a combination of bad carbs and fats.

For many years we have struggled to reduce the amount of fat in our diets, and yet the population has continued to become overweight. What manufacturers do when they take the fat out of the food is compensate by adding more sugar. So of course it makes no difference that it now has a 'low fat' label. The carbohydrate will make you put on weight much the same.

By controlling the chemicals in your brain, your body can guide you to those types of combinations that will best allow you to put on weight. Just look at any fast food. I guarantee you that in every case, it's a combination of fat and bad carbs. The phenomenal growth of these types of food is not only because of aggressive and clever marketing, but also the body's love of absorbing energy. People are easily caught in the trap of lack of exercise and a high energy diet. As the weight increases, the person becomes more sedentary because of the sheer physical effort required to carry the extra weight and the need to compensate with high sugar/fat foods goes up. As the years go by, the person eventually reaches a point of equilibrium, where the amount of food going in equals the amount of energy coming out. The energy levels become low and the person now only eats small amounts, but never loses weight.

We have found in these cases that when people are caught in the situation, after following *GI Feel Good: Health and Weight Loss*, the patients are capable of dropping dramatic amounts of weight in the first few weeks. I think from memory 8 kilos (16 pounds) in a couple of weeks is the record. It seems the change in circumstances catches the body by surprise and it readily gives up the weight. Normally the weight loss will eventually stabilise, and continue to come off at the usual 500g to 1 kilo (1 to 2 pounds) a week.

CHAPTER 4

Frequently asked questions

When starting something totally new, there is always going to be some questions. Here is a random selection of the most common questions that beginners usually ask. Just remember that if your question is not here then try our website forum where there are literally thousands of people's questions and answers.

How come I can eat cheese and cream but can't have milk or yoghurt?

Originally we included milk and yoghurt in our first book *Sugar Science*, and for the most part few people had any problems, but gradually over time some people reported to us that they were not getting the desired effect. The only reason we could see was that milk and yoghurt (which is by the way, fermented milk) contain lactose. Lactose is a sugar like glucose, sucrose, fructose and so on – being a sugar, we could only conclude the lactose must have an effect on the glycogen in the liver and gradually over time cause some people to flounder.

In recent years there has been a few milks and yoghurts that have come on the market that have a GI around 30, so technically it should be fine with moderate carb breakfasts. You are more than welcome to give them a try but you will probably find that you are not losing the desired weight and if that's the case then, from experience, this would be one of the first things to take out. I personally never drink milk and, from what I understand, cows don't either. Only *baby* cows drink milk. Why? Because it's full of growth hormones, sugars and fats. More compelling is a study, conducted here in Australia, that made a connection between tumour growth and the growth hormone in milk – look it up on the Internet if you want more information. For me, that was pretty good reason to get over drinking milk.

Another thing that you may come across is 'lactose-free' milk. All the manufacturers have done is take the lactose and convert it into glucose or galactose. The reason they do this is because some people are lactose intolerant. Actually it's because milk contains a protein that irritates the lining of the gut and causes inflammation. One way or the other changing it into glucose means it cannot be included, so forget about this one as well. In my opinion it's much easier to just 'bite the bullet' and get used to the taste of the soymilk.

Why can you eat cheese and not drink milk? Again it's to do with the lactose. The more lactose something contains the more of the problem it's going to be. Think of it as a scale, with milk at one end and hard cheese down the other. Cheese is mostly fat and a little bit of lactose: milk on the other hand is mostly lactose and a little bit of fat. When eating the cheese there is hardly any lactose and the GI of cheese is often so low its GI is undetectable. Milk we already know about and you will notice that the GI for full cream milk has a lower GI than skimmed milk. Why is that? The reason for this is because when fat is included, it takes longer to digest and as a result, slows down the digestion giving the food a *slightly* lower GI. Before you get any ideas and start adding butter to your apple juice, don't bother! You will bring yourself undone. Just "swim between the flags" and you will be fine.*

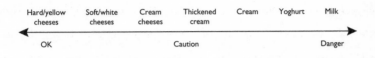

Now, think of the scale above with cheese at one end and milk at the other – you would have the hard cheeses, then soft cheeses next, then creamed cheeses. Towards the middle you would have the creams and then as you move further along start getting your yoghurts and then full cream milk, and eventually the skinny milks and so on at the opposite end. For example, some of the recipes in this book call for some cream. That's fine because it's with a protein meal that has fat – it's going to drag the cream back in to the safety zone. However some people, believe it or not, will just eat cream on its own 'because the book says you can eat cream'. This would not be a good idea because

* On Australian surf beaches flags are put out by the surf life savers to show where it is safe to swim.

the lactose in the cream will start to ruin your progress, however in a meal it's not as much of a problem but the quantities do matter. So a little cream is fine as per the recipe, whereas drowning food in cream may be a problem.

Can I eat fruit after my meal?

Fruit has a moderate glycemic index, and therefore can only be combined with other moderate carbohydrates. If you ate fruit at the end of a protein meal, namely one that contains fat, then, as I have described earlier, that meal would become fattening as a result. The answer is if you have a carbohydrate meal, you can include fruit, but with a protein meal you cannot. There is something quite unique about fruit. When you eat proteins the stomach becomes more acidic. When you eat carbohydrates the stomach becomes more alkaline. The funny thing about fruit is that it requires somewhere in between an acid and alkaline environment to be digested.

When you combine it with other foods it has the effect of disrupting the digestive process to some degree. That is why fruit is best eaten on an empty stomach. I normally eat fruit first thing in the morning, before eating the other carbohydrates that constitute my breakfast, like cereal for example. I then tend to forget about it for the rest of the day.

What can I have on my cereal in the morning?

Soymilk is what we advise. Cow's milk can make life difficult as I mentioned earlier. With soymilk one needs to read the information on the box first, and it is best to purchase the one with the lowest amount of sugar. You must try to find the 'malt-free' variety. We have always bought Australia's Own malt-free, for example. If you can't get this brand then you are looking for the one with the least amount of sugar per 100g. Less than 1g is best. Australia's Own is 0.4g per 100 for example. Soymilk is an acquired taste and I think most of the ones I have tried, with the exception of Australia's Own, taste awful. Give it a try.

Can I drink alcohol?

Alcohol, by and large, contains a lot of carbohydrate. Even if you include red wine, which contains very little sugar, it becomes difficult to lose weight. Some people have reported that they still managed to drink the occasional wine and not have it affect them, but what usually happens eventually is the weight loss stalls at some point, so once again, stay between the flags and swear off the booze while you are in the weight loss phase. Put the money you save to buying nice food and the new outfit.

Are all fruits okay or should some be avoided?

Originally we included all fruits, but over time we have found that fruits like banana, watermelon and grapes are just too high in the GI and should be avoided. As for strawberries, rock-melon and kiwi fruit, approach them with caution and just don't go overboard as they can affect your glycogen levels and cause you to plateau. When considering a certain fruit, check the GI in the tables at the back of the book or go to the website www.glycemic-index.com. The lower the GI the better and as with all the moderate carbs, just don't go overboard, use them in moderation.

Another thing that you need to be aware of is quite often people will conclude that because certain fruits are okay, then the fruit juice must be okay as well. Unfortunately when you vitamise the fruit into juice, you are liberating the carbohydrate in the fruit and making it easier to absorb, so you have to be careful with apple juice, blackcurrent juice, cranberry juice and the like. It can make life difficult.

Can I have artificial sweeteners?

There has been much debate on this subject. Originally, when I wrote my first book, I said 'yes'. Diabetics used them; artificial sweeteners didn't affect BSLs (so I thought) and my conclusion was 'why not?'. I thought that making a point about them being bad for your health would be enough to discourage people from using them.

There were two things I was unaware of. First, there is an incredible variety of artificial sweeteners on the market and to my surprise I found out some affected the BSLs almost the same as sugar did, some even more than sugar. Manufacturers had managed to slip past the sugar-free safety net by simply changing the sugar into maltose or glucose so technically it wasn't sugar and could be called 'sugar-free'. The other thing that we didn't anticipate is that some people become addicted to using them. When I explained in my first book that some artificial sweeteners were carcinogenic, in my mind I thought that that should be enough to persuade people from using them. I was wrong. Some people are deeply addicted to using them. Diet colas are a good example. I have met that many people who in their own words are hooked on drinking diet colas. It's a pity because if you look up artificial sweeteners like phenylalanine and aspartame on the Internet, you get a load of the websites warning people of the hidden dangers and the side effects.

If you visit our website forum, you will also see that many 'newbies' (new people) ask about artificial sweeteners. Unfortunately it takes up a disproportionate amount of resources to have to keep answering the same question.

For many years we said 'We don't recommend it', not simply from the health side of it, but also because many people had reported that they were not achieving the desired results while using them. Then we came across something new – Cephalic Phase Insulin Response (CPIR). Researchers had discovered that when you taste something sweet, your brain signals the pancreas to release insulin in preparation for the rise in the BSL even before it has had time to reached the gut. This shed light on the fact that some people who were using artificial sweeteners were still having difficulty getting their weight or cholesterol down. Even though the food they ate had a low GI, the sweet 'sugar-free' lolly or drink they followed it up with was making the body release insulin and absorb the fats regardless.

So why did the people have them in the first place? The answer is simple – people get addicted to sweet things. Why have something sweet when it offers no nutrition, does nothing for your body and is bad for your health? There can only be one answer: it's psychological. People believe that if they don't taste something sweet, there're not happy, when in actual fact it's the brain releasing chemicals to make you feel that way, that's all. Unfortunately for me that's not a good enough reason to crave sweet food, and when I think about it,

I actually find I get unhappy when I taste something really sweet because I know the effect it will have on me. I'll probably end up wanting to overeat. There's a chemical in my brain making me feel that way. I don't really want it, I don't need to eat it, but my kooky 'grey matter' with its built-in primordial mechanism and pleasure centres has another agenda. The fact is I know I'm not starving, I know I'm not lost in the bush trying to survive, so for now I'm going to ignore that instinct and focus on something more important like my health and not being controlled by food. So the official answer is 'Stay between the flags and don't use artificial sweeteners'.

Should I take vitamins and minerals?

The idea is that you get your vitamins and minerals from having a balanced diet. That being said I have always taken vitamins since childhood so it's a matter of preference. If you are buying a supplement then make sure that sugar or starch isn't listed as an ingredient. You would be surprised what you find when you read the label. Just as an aside it is interesting to note that Recommended Daily Allowance (RDA) was actually something that was determined at the start of World War II when England, fearing being blockaded by the Germans, wanted to know what the absolute minimum amount of vitamins people could take without developing illnesses like scurvy. The RDA means you are only getting the minimum amount of nutrients without becoming ill. Personally vitamin and mineral supplements are much of a muchness and I think whatever brand you buy comes down to personal preference.

Is it anything like the Atkins diet?

Roberts Atkins was a cardiologist who, in the 1960s, was trying to find a way to lose weight. After reading reports about the relationship between carbohydrate, insulin and fat, he pioneered a formula for controlling weight by controlling insulin. Originally he just relyed on a pure protein diet. This was long before the GI and originally he just had people lose weight by eating meat. As time went by he eventually worked out exactly how much carbohydrate you could give a person and still have them lose weight. So by restricting the person's intake of carbohydrates and getting them to eat lots of protein he was able to achieve good results with weight loss. This method is now known as 'the Atkins Diet'. Unfortunately for Dr Atkins, restricting the amount of carbohydrate and getting people to eat lots of meat became the biggest criticism of his method and many people attacked him for promoting an 'unhealthy diet'.

When a person is on a low GI diet, the amount of carbohydrate doesn't matter. What does matter is the type. As a result one can have as much of the low GI carbohydrate with their protein meals as they like. It doesn't matter and, as I said before, be moderate with the moderate carbs, and you should get good results.

So although *GI Feel Good: Health and Weight Loss* and the Atkins diet both focus on carbs, the main difference is that a *GI Feel Good: Health and Weight Loss* doesn't restrict the intake of carbohydrate. The results are similar, but patients who have tried both often say that my version is much easier to follow.

Interestingly enough, the late Dr Atkins was aware of the GI but felt that it was nothing more than a 'useful reference' and didn't see the need to reinvent his program because of it.

I'm not getting much support from friends and family.

People don't like it when they see others doing something that they can't do themselves, like losing weight and getting healthy, so all they can do is criticise in an attempt to get control of the situation. The answer is simple: let the results speak for themselves and that should put an end to it. People can make out that they are looking out for your best interest but actually they can be just undermining you. It's time to shine and get on with the job at hand. Choose your friends wisely and look for support from those genuinely willing to give it. Our website forum is a good source of inspiration.

How long do I keep doing this?

On the website we have what's called a Body Mass Indicator (BMI). You just plug in your height, weight and age and it gives you a figure. Compare that figure with a chart and it gives you a fairly good idea if your weight is in the normal range or not. I think if you need to lose weight, then the first step would be to get a good idea of what your normal weight range should be.

Being overweight is very much like being in debt, you've borrowed money that you don't actually have and eventually have to pay back. With the body, being overweight is when you have 'borrowed' more energy from your food than your body actually needs and to get rid of it you have to stop

216

borrowing and let the body gradually use it up. For some people losing weight can be very abstract but paying back money is far more concrete. Sometimes it helps to use a metaphor like this, to get a grip on the situation. Just think of losing weight like paying off a debt. The more weight that comes off, the closer you are to being free of the burden.

The average person, while following our formula, will burn up roughly half to one kilo (1 to 2 pounds) of body fat a week. If you take the number of kilos you need to lose and make it a week or so for each, you will have a rough idea of the time you can expect to be doing everything 'by the book'. We also provide a service where we will track what you have been eating and your progress and give you advice on getting the best results each week. Again, it's all on our website, www.glycemic-index.com.

People usually have a goal and they just keep going until they have reached it and are happy with their weight. After that they usually have a splurge, feel really sick afterwards and then go back to following the maintenance side of the book. If you find you are getting 'kilo creep', or in other words, the weight is starting to go up again, then do things strictly for a while until you are back to your comfortable weight again. There's no harm in doing this, the only harm is emotionally when you find your new slacks are starting to look a bit tight.

Newbies like to play around but if they are not careful can fall back into the habit of eating the way they did before and soon find themselves back to square one. The longer people have been following it the harder it is to go to your old ways. You don't need to believe me – if you stay with it long enough, you will find out for yourself. Your body won't let you do it to yourself. Why? Because you have both known what it was like to be sugar-free, and it's hard to forget how good you felt. That's why I called the book '*GI Feel Good*' – it's because that's what most people say.

We all have to live by our choices and no one will be there to stop you from trying to undo all the good work you have done already. Only you have the power, but when you understand why it is that you are avoiding the bad carbs and other sweet things, it becomes a lot easier to make that decision.

I have a really slow metabolism.

Often I have heard people say this to me and for a very long time all I could tell them was eating more actually stimulates the metabolism and speeds it up (another pleasing feature of the book). But it was with great interest when I read a report a number of years ago that tested the theory about overweight people having slow metabolisms. What the study had discovered was that overweight people actually had faster metabolisms than average. The report found that carrying the extra weight made the body work harder. The result was the higher metabolism. When you think about it, carrying something heavy always requires more energy. If you have ever carried a backpack, and for most people around 30 kilos (60 pounds) is going to be maximum permissible weight before performance starts to drop, you will appreciate how much extra effort is required. I have had patients lose over 45 kilos (90 pounds). The heaviest backpack that I had ever carried was 33 kilos (66 pounds) and I could not contemplate carrying 45 kilos (90 pounds) without great difficulty and exertion.

If you ever want a wake-up call as to how much weight you've already lost, at the supermarket grab the equivalent weight in bags of oranges and then wander around with them in your arms, saying to yourself 'Crikey! This is what I used to carry around every day'. I always find it's refreshing to have something tangible to compare the weight with. It's a sobering thought. You don't have to say crikey by the way, it's just a suggestion. Use your own cultural expletive if you like (there's a list in the back of the book).

My friend is really skinny and they can eat whatever they like.

Remember how I explained that if the energy input is less than energy output, people lose weight? If the amount of energy that the person is putting into their bodies equals the amount of energy that they are putting out then their weight will stay the same. Some people burn the energy quicker, some people are under a lot of stress, some people do physical labour for a living – these kinds of people use up all the energy in their diet every day. That's why they can even struggle to maintain the weight and when stressed, lose weight. If you have ever bemoaned the fact that when you were young you could eat what ever you liked and now you can't, its because when you were young your hormone levels were different and you were more active. You have to make adjustment for your age. Even children who don't exercise can put on weight just like adults.

Don't forget also that people who smoke can also be quite skinny. The main reason behind this is the smoking dehydrates the body so there is less fluid. The person will always look skinnier. Ever wondered why so many models smoke? What happens is when the person stops, they can suddenly put on weight. One reason is because the person is rehydrating and the other is because they replace the oral fixation satisfied with cigarettes with food. Believe it or not, I have even met women who are too frightened to stop smoking for fear of putting on weight. The rebounding weight is only transient and following the book will sort that out.

Why doesn't quantity matter?

Quantity only matters when eating the moderate carbs. Remember the motto is 'eat moderate carbs in moderation'. Why? Simply because when eating the moderate carbs your body is getting energy from the carbohydrate – if you eat too much, you can create a surplus which your body can start embezzling. The surplus goes to the liver and gradually the liver starts to fill up again with glycogen. When this happens your body is no longer using the fat as a source of energy, but that rather the glycogen in the liver and your weight loss stops. This is the only reason why the people plateau.

When it comes to the protein meals, and the good GI carbs, there is no risk of having a surplus of energy from the carbohydrates. In this context you can eat as much as you feel like and that is the reason why the quantity doesn't matter. If you think of the food going into the body is like putting vegetables into a food processor, you can force more in and fill the whole shoot, but the motor still runs at roughly the same speed and still spits out the vegetables at the same rate. So if you were trying to raise your blood sugar levels by just eating the low GI carbs like tomato, mushrooms and salad and so on, then the more and more you shoved into your mouth would not change the speed your digestion processes it. Because it can only be broken down at the same rate, the amount of the glucose being released into your blood would remain low. So you can sit down to a large protein meal and as long as you are still using the low GI 'good' carbs then it doesn't matter how much of the protein your eating.

If I keep going is there any danger of becoming too thin?

I know for a lot of people being slim is like a dream. Believe me I have seen many people become slim and healthy and achieve their dreams. It's very emotional. But have I ever seen someone who is getting dangerously skinny? No. Not even the models I have seen as patients. The reason is when you are following my book, you are eating very well and your body is simply using the fat it has in storage for energy. Because you are only burning up fat, there's no risk of losing the muscle mass and becoming skeletal. What you can expect is to reach a weight that is ideal for you. That's why we have the BMI chart on our website, so you can get an idea of your ideal weight. There is a point for every person when they're not carrying the extra weight. So even though you can become slim you will never be skeletal.

What do I do when I want a snack?

If you eat a reasonable amount at each meal, then the need for snacking disappears. Every so often, you find that you're getting hungry and there still is a little time before the next meal, the best thing to do is to eat something that is going to be okay with the next meal. So for example if the next meal is a protein meal, then eating some cheese before the meal is fine. If the meal is a carb meal then having some dried fruit beforehand will be okay as well. Remember that you still have to think about the time windows if you are swapping from one meal type to another. If you had a carb breakfast and then three hours later decided to have some fruit before your protein lunch, as you know, you would have extended the time window by a further three hours. (Read the section on 'time windows' again if you are unsure.) The easiest way to avoid snacking is just to eat more for breakfast and lunch and dinner. Eating at regular intervals also gives your digestion the chance to have a break in between. Constantly grazing doesn't give the digestion time-out and keeps it constantly working, which eventually makes it sluggish.

I don't seem to be as regular

It is not unusual for some people to find in the initial stages that they are not as regular in the beginning. This is for two reasons. Firstly you are most likely eating more protein than before, which is a little harder to digest and slows things down. The other reason is because the gas is no longer in the intestines like before. You may have noticed that you are no longer bloated – the bloating acts like pressure in a champagne bottle trying to push out the cork. Without the pressure, the large intestine has to use its muscles to massage the food along and they may have become weak and need a little time to catch up again. So in the first couple of weeks you may not be as regular as before. Just add a little more fibre to your muesli and after a little while you should find things will be back to normal.

Should I eat carbs at night or should I eat protein?

You will find that the eating protein in the evening will give you better results. The reason is because the body scavenges for energy when you are asleep. If you eat carbohydrates at night before going to bed your body will use the available fuel in the carbohydrates to replenish its energy reserves. If you eat protein your body will not be able to get the reserves from the meal and instead will draw more heavily on the fat stored in the body. So generally speaking it's better to eat protein at night if you are really trying to do everything right.

I am taking medication. Does that matter?

Some medications do affect your weight. Cortisone for example causes fluid retention as well as other steroids. Birth control pills and synthetic oestrogens like HRT can also cause fluid retention. This can be a contributing factor when you are trying to get the weight down and unfortunately there may not be a lot you can do about it. Best to talk to your doctor and see if they have any suggestions.

How much exercise do I need to do?

Exercise is an essential part of daily activity, however it is not essential as far as this book goes. As you can see the only exercise you really need to do is to exercise proper judgement when deciding what to eat for each meal. One of the things that I always find unfortunate is seeing overweight people jogging to lose weight. 'If they only had a copy of the book,' I would often think, 'then the whole job would be so much easier'. (Chérie has actually had to caution me about hurling copies from the car window.) The sad part is that the person has already overtaxed themselves by not eating correctly, and now they are putting an even greater strain on their bodies by trying to burn it off. With the GI, it is much easier to lose the weight first and then, as you get closer to your desired weight, begin getting into shape in the gym or on the track.

After teaching martial arts for almost twenty years, I am no stranger to daily exercise. The Chinese believe that anything that requires you to break into a light sweat is sufficient exercise. Tai Chi, walking, rebounding, swimming, Pilates, yoga or cycling are all good choices, and can be enjoyed regardless of your age.

Having said that, I have also met a great many people who have chosen to follow my book and go to the gym. What happens usually in this scenario is that the weight seems to come off quicker, but it really depends on how much extra effort the person puts into it. If this is the way you would like to go about it then 'more power to you', but unless there is some particular reason why you need it to come off faster, then the fact of the matter is, you will achieve the same results, without flogging yourself around the block. You can save your time and put your money towards the gym membership when you have eventually lost the weight and want to tone up.

I have selected a range of exercise that I believe that

have unique health benefits and if you like, you can read more about these activities in the appendices section at the back of the book.

If I come off the rails, how should I get back on track?

If, for some nefarious reason, you had discovered that the forces of darkness have been arrayed against you and somehow managed to undermine your best efforts (because let's face it, how else would you possibly come off the rails?), my advice is the following day, when you are facing your sugar cravings all over again, just eat fruit for a meal. Your body will think its getting sugar when in actual fact it is not doing any harm and this can get things going again. Rather than beating yourself up, redouble your efforts and try to learn from the experience, thinking in particular about where you went wrong and see if you can develop a better strategy for the future.

I've reached a plateau

I thought about having a sealed section which read 'Open only in case of emergency' – inside it would say 'Relax'.

It is normal from time to time for the weight loss graph to flatten out – there can be a variety of factors. Time of month and its attendant fluid retention, what's already in your digestive track that has yet to come out and eating salty things can make you retain fluid – even colder weather can slow you down. So there's no need to have to panic, it will get started again when it's ready and not everyone is going to lose weight at the same rate. For some it's slower, but the main thing is they are still losing weight and that's the main thing.

Remember that you can still be going down in size without losing weight, so that's why it's a good idea to have a tape measure.

If you find that you have stayed the same weight or size for a while and 'seem' to be doing everything right and following the advice you have been given, then normally the advice I give is 'try eating more protein meals to get things going again'. The explanation is a little complex but even when doing everything 'by the book' sometimes your body can still get some 'mileage' from the moderate carbs that you have been eating. Occasionally the glycogen in the liver can go from being empty to slowly getting topped up again over time. If your body discovers that you have energy reserves in the liver, it switches back to the liver for fuel and leaves the reserves found on your hips and thighs. Eating protein has the effect of driving down the glycogen levels again and restarting the weight loss.

If you have tried this and are still not making progress then you have to look once again at what you're putting in your mouth. Occasionally a person will report this to us and what we ask them to do is submit a diary of what they have been eating for the past few weeks and from there, we can see if they have been doing things right. Believe it or not in spite of people's protestations when it gets to this stage there has not been a single submission that has not revealed the problem. Often it's artificial sweeteners, in spite of the advice, or milk, just little things like this that can be the culprit. As I mentioned earlier we provide a service to track what you have been eating and offer advice from the sidelines, this should be enough for you to avoid any pitfalls. So if you do find things are not going as smoothly as possible always go back to what you have been eating and make sure you are following the advice and not being a little too generous with the moderate carbs. Try eating more protein to begin with and if that still doesn't work get in touch with our centre. The details for the online support are in the back of the book.

Will I be able to stay on this indefinitely?

Why not? Following my book is very much like following mainstream eating. That is of course, if your eating includes many tasty and the occasional gourmet dishes. Most people, having become proficient with the process, preferred to stay with it, only occasionally having the odd meal that doesn't fit within the guidelines. The long-term advice to any person is that eating high-protein all the time may not be the best idea and you want to be sure that you are getting plenty of fibre from grains, vegetables and so on in the diet. You can include as many of the right carbohydrates in your diet as you choose and there should be no reason to constantly rely on high-protein. Of course in the initial stages when wanting to lose the weight, eating more protein is preferable, but to keep eating high-protein indefinitely would be unnecessary. Personally, I find that I eat more of the protein meals in general, so what I try to do is garnish the protein meals with plenty of the vegetables, as I find that this is more of a balanced approach for long-term health.

What is ketosis?

'Okay sit up straight, it's thinking cap time again'. Another amazing thing that your body does, is when you eat protein with low GI carbs, it makes up for the lack of energy in the carbs, by burning your fat reserves. This is called ketolypolysis (kee-toe-ly-po-ly-sis) or ketosis for short. What this means is eating protein makes your body burn fat. It sounds too good to be true. If we all just ate protein we would all lose weight and this was exactly what Robert Atkins discovered, however he also discovered that there was one small problem with this. If a person just ate meat exclusively then their blood would eventually become so acidic that it would start to damage the liver and the kidneys. This is called ketoacidosis and is an undesirable consequence of taking this action.

Believe it or not I have had patients come to me and tell me that they had been told by their personal trainer or some such that this is what they must do to lose weight. Naturally they are wrong. Eating carbohydrates stops this from ever happening and when following my book you can eat as much of the low GI carbs as you like and eat plenty of protein if you prefer and never worry about this. Of course it's not necessary to just strictly eat only the 'protein meal' that we have in the book. Speaking from experience, just eating high-protein does get a bit much after awhile. What I normally do is have Chérie's untoasted muesli with fresh fruit for breakfast, then for lunch I usually have protein, because I like my main meal at lunchtime and it fills me up so I don't get hungry until dinner. I normally work until dinner. At dinnertime I will have something smaller. Sometimes it's a carb meal like pasta, sometimes a protein meal – again, I am not too fussed. Sometimes I don't eat again until breakfast.

I find that this works for me, but you may like to do it differently. A good rule of thumb is your blood type. O blood-types prefer protein, which is me, A blood-types prefer carbs, B's are a bit of both and so are ABs. There is a great book about blood types and diet called *Eat Right for Your Blood Type*. For example, it's not unusual for an O blood-type, the most common, to come and see me because they have decided to become a vegetarian, only to discover sometime later down the track their energy levels are through the floor. O blood-type vegetarians usually hit the wall in their early thirties and by the time they see me it's usually the end of being a vegetarian. Conversely A blood-types who have been vegetarian for many years may seldom have problems with their diet – that's not to say they won't develop problems, it's just that they usually suffer from different things. You will have to experiment to find out what's best for you.

What do I eat when I go out for a meal?

Just about every menu will include at least three dishes that fall within the guidelines. A steak, piece of chicken or grilled fish for example. If this is not the case, it is very simple to have the kitchen omit one or two ingredients to make the meal okay. One technique for avoiding certain ingredients is to feign food allergies. A useful technique, for example, is to say something like 'Oh my specialist has told me that I am allergic to starch'. People, for some reason, will not question expert advice on another person's health. This is usually enough to fob off unwanted attention and is a simple solution, rather than explaining that you are trying to follow a diet. This always requires some explanation, and the intricacies of knowledge such as this can be lost on the uninitiated.

Will I ever be able to eat these types of foods again?

Up to you really, once you have the knowledge it's yours to do with as you see fit. What you will probably discover is the bad carbs still taste good to you but the feeling of wellbeing that you have will suit you better. You will find it harder to have those binges like you did before. Realistically, you should forget about the things that are not good for you. Once you have a firm understanding of this knowledge, then the art of looking after your health is yours. Should you find yourself eating those things that you know will make you put on weight, then you know the easiest way to lose it again.

I can't do it because (make up your own excuse and insert here) . . .

Pat Farmer is an Australian Ultra Marathon runner who, in the year 2000, ran right around the coastline of Australia, including Tasmania! Think about it. To describe it as an incredible achievement would be an understatement. After arriving back in Sydney, he summarised his achievement with these words:

'When you really want to do something, in your heart of hearts, you will find a way, but if you don't want to do something, you will find an excuse.'

Pat, if you ever read this, I couldn't agree with you more. People who have made remarkable changes, to themselves and their lives, have put aside their excuses and 'found a way' to achieve their goals. When it really comes down to doing some-

230

thing, you end up just getting on with it. When you think back over your life, the times when you have achieved a personal milestone has always come with resolution and commitment. I thought Pat put it better than I ever could. Don't try to find excuses. Just get on with it. Do it and achieve your goals. Study the book, understand it, then off you go – you will be surprised at the difference it will make to you and your life, and you may just end up experiencing yourself in a totally new way.

If this is so great, why hasn't my doctor or dietician heard about it?

Good question. As mentioned earlier a recent survey on the US website, www.abcnews.com, asked 'Out of low calorie, low fat or low carb, which was the most successful diet?' Several thousand people responded and low carb polled at around 60%, the highest response. So one could say that it is the most popular diet in the US at the moment. The glycemic index has been around for more than twenty years, and low carb recipes for the past five, so I often wonder why professional people still struggle to come to grips with it. Part of the reason, I believe, is that many would have to admit that they have been giving people the wrong information for many years, and you know what people are like when it comes to admitting they are wrong. Occasionally doctors who have read my book will recommend it to their patients – I am always grateful for the endorsement and support. We have to get the message out there somehow even though there are those who would prefer it that you knew nothing of this.

I knew back in 1995 that the glycemic index was going to totally change the way we think, and I am glad to say that I was right. Every day I have people telling me how much weight they have lost, how their lives have changed, they feel better, haven't got a cholesterol problem, they're pregnant and so on. We are very glad that these changes are filtering out into the mainstream. More recently the GI value of some foods has been included on the packaging.

Swim between the flags

In the early days we would receive regular phone calls and emails from people asking questions. Eventually it was taking up a disproportionate amount of time answering these same questions each day, so I decided that the website should have a forum with a dedicated person answering people's inquiries. Today the forum has become a very useful resource for beginners and veterans alike. There's mutual support from others who are discovering the GI as well as some very useful insights and moving stories. The forum's Oracle 'Kelly' is also on hand to answer some of the tricky questions. If you visit the forum you will discover it's open 24/7 with more than 2000 questions and replies. We also provide an online service where we review what you are eating on a week-to-week basis and coach you from the sidelines. It's all there on the website: www.glycemic-index.com.

I have often used a metaphor of surf lifesaving when learning how to use the GI. When you visit a surf beach you will find that volunteers are giving up their time to be there for you. The flags are there to guide you and if you have never been to a surf beach, the idea is to swim between the flags because it's safe to do so – outside of that and you can get into difficulty, start to struggle and someone may have to come and pull you out. Now the vast majority of people 'swim between the flags' and never have any problems, but there are always those who may not be very strong swimmers and can need a helping hand from time to time. Our website offers tremendous support.

In spite of this there are those who always want to test the boundaries and can often manipulate advice to suit themselves. If you want to be successful, follow our advice and swim between the flags, that way you will avoid difficulty.

CHAPTER 5

Low GI and the healthy kiddie

Overweight children have become an emerging problem over the last ten years. There has been much debate as to why our youth are becoming so overweight, but when you read statistics that in Australia, one in four children are overweight, and one in five obese, you have to sit up and take notice. For me the alarm bells started ringing long ago when I started seeing children as young as seven developing adult diseases. Children as young as this had developed arteriosclerosis and mature onset diabetes, diseases normally seen in middle-aged people. We are facing an enormous epidemic of illness in the young, which will play itself out over the next 10 to 20 years with disastrous consequences. We must act now.

Often parents approach me, to see if my book would be suitable for their children. Naturally there is no problem with children following a low GI diet, the only thing that they are not getting is the *excess* energy from the food. However from my experience, parents need only cut out the bad carbs to get the desired result. Children burn much more energy than adults, and by reducing the surplus of energy they're receiving, it becomes very easy for them to lose the weight again. More about this later, I would like to get out the soapbox for the moment.

I don't need to tell you that children's diets are high in sugar. One needs only to look at how much of it is in the contents of products that are advertised as 'healthy for children' – it's staggering. If you want jaw-dropping examples of diet madness, look at the US. Children not only have access to a wide variety of 'junk food' in their canteens, they also have access to Pizza Hut, Burger King and McDonald's in the actual school! In some schools children can even drink Coke and Dr Pepper in class. How could parents permit such questionable choices, you may wonder? The answer is simple. To the parents this is the type of food that they as children where brought up on and is considered normal. Unfortunately the evidence is all too obvious. The obesity epidemic in the US is out of control.

In the US, drink companies offer incentives to schools to sell more of their products. If the school reaches a certain quota of soft drinks each year they receive a cash bonus. Companies also pay to advertise their products in the children's schoolbooks, diaries and classrooms. One school even had the company's trademark painted on the roof of one of its buildings, so that low-flying aircraft landing at a nearby airport could see who sponsored the school. There are always things that we say could not happen here. We have been wrong in the past about many of them, but we must draw a line in the sand when it comes to the health of our children. If you are a parent you have a moral obligation to take care of the health of your child. Naturally I don't wish to preach the obvious, but long after you have gone your children will be there without you – one of the lasting legacies that they will carry with them is their health. It is not that difficult, simply helping children to make the right choices when they are young can lead them to healthy eating patterns that will last with the rest of their lives. They in turn will pass this behaviour on to their children and so on and so on.

Of course I realise that you have been bombarded with similar messages for many years, but the problem is there is no concrete advice on what to actually do. So allow me to give you some guidance.

If your child is not overweight, I wouldn't be too critical of the diet – usually in this situation, the child is very active and is burning up the energy just as nature intended. I would just be aware of how much sugar is in the actual diet, simply because sugar has no nutritional value, and if it's this empty carbohydrate that's bulking out the diet, then this may be problematic.

A very interesting result from one of the many studies into childhood obesity was that overweight children were often thought of as being overnourished. As it turned out many over-weight children are in fact undernourished! The food that they are getting, although high in sugar and fat, has very little nutritional value and as a result children's growth is stunted, bones are brittle, eyesight and teeth weak. Occasionally I will see a child who is overweight but unusually small for their age. Often the reason for this they are undernourished and failing to develop properly.

If your child is overweight, then, as I described earlier, simply taking the 'bad carbs' out of the diet usually allows the child to burn up the excess energy. And they will tend to lose the puppy fat. A low GI diet contains grains, vegetables, meats, fish, oils, eggs and cheese. There is no nutritionist in the country who would argue that that is not healthy. The simple fact that they are not receiving the high GI food only means they are not getting a surplus of energy.

If the child is morbidly obese, which means that they are in danger of developing disease from being overweight, then things have to be done strictly by the book. Grandparents and other children's parents who have access to your child's diet must cooperate with what you wish your child to eat. There is no point getting everything right at home only for the child to get the wrong food when they visit somewhere else. Again, this is a problem that only you can solve.

Having the child understand why their diet has to change can help them understand more about what they are eating. When it becomes a question of motivation over education, always choose education, because when someone understands what they are doing, then they will motivate themselves. Often parents have described their children's proactive behaviour upon understanding the necessities. Children become very particular about what they are eating when they understand the benefits. Set milestones and achievable goals for the child. They can be rewarded with things other than food for making it to a particular milestone. Clothes, gadgets, movies and outings are all examples of rewards for the child that don't involve food. Making food a reward is a very big mistake in my opinion, simply because many adults I have dealt with view food as a

238

reward also. When you are the person who is giving the reward as well as receiving the reward it becomes quite difficult not to continually reward yourself with food. What generally happens is the person continually finds reasons for rewarding themselves or 'comforting' themselves with food. Inevitably food becomes a focal point in their life, and as a result these treats become a vicious circle.

Like everything, this pattern of behaviour has its origins in childhood. While on the subject, as I have mentioned before, making children clean their plates before leaving the table is another problem. You may remember as a child having to sit at the table and forcing yourself to fight back the waves of nausea as you try to eat something Mum has boiled to destruction. As unpleasant as this may seem, besides forcing you to eat Brussels sprouts (which we all know was created in a laboratory by some crazed neo-fascists bent on destroying generation X), simply ask yourself 'how often do you eat Brussels sprouts now'? If your answer is 'not at all', then you will realise that this was an entirely wasted exercise. If you look beyond my questionable conspiracy theory, forcing a child to eat teaches them to override your body's signal to stop eating. A part of compulsive eating is ignoring your body's signals to stop. Again this is something that begins in early childhood behaviour and its origins begin at the table.

While on the subject of overweight children, as I said earlier, there has been numerous studies done by various government elements. One report I found interesting felt that the calorie intake of children had changed little over the past ten years, however the amount of exercise each day had fallen dramatically. They argued that obesity epidemic is a result of lack of daily activity, rather then increase eating. I felt this was worth mentioning and is it has become quite apparent that children tend to spend more time in front of television watching cartoons or playing video games, rather then running around outside playing. Again drawing from childhood experience, I can vividly remember my mother begging us to come inside for dinner. With daylight savings in full effect and not getting dark until nine pm, this meant more playtime after school for children in my street. Moreover I remember the long walk home from the tram stop carrying an increasingly heavy school bag. The thought of being driven each day was the stuff of fantasy. I know there's such a thing as stranger danger, and we have to protect our children, but there must be a balance between providing a safe environment for them and insulating the children unnecessarily. Schools need to be more proactive about sports. Some parents had even complained to me that the school doesn't allow the children to play on the monkey bars for fear of public liability. You may not believe that in some schools even running is not allowed, for the same reason. Now come on, running? No stretch of imagination could describe where I went as a 'tough' school. Let's face it, you could have a reign of terror with a balloon on a stick if you wanted to but we were still allowed to run around.

Like it or not we are faced with a problem from which the long-term consequences are very grave indeed. An overweight child very often becomes an overweight adult and, as I identified early on in the piece, being overweight is not necessarily benign. Besides the risk of heart disease and diabetes, poor self-esteem and self-image is crippling to young people becoming adolescent.

Another interesting study done here in Australia dealt with taking overweight children and instead of focusing solely on diet, they encouraged the children to exercise each day using exercise equipment. The equipment involved the type of apparatus that you see in most gymnasiums that are designed to increase strength by using weights. Normally overweight people are encouraged to do cardiovascular exercises that involve walking machines and exercise bikes in an attempt to 'burn off' the excess weight. It seems counterintuitive to encourage overweight people to try to increase muscle strength while still carrying the extra weight. What researchers discovered was the children did not lose any remarkable amount of weight, but they did becomes stronger and developed muscular fitness. As a result, they became disinclined to sit idly in front of television, and more inclined to include physical activity in their play. Being stronger, they were able to do more things and the increase in physical activity resulted in the children burning up more of the excess fat.

Going to gymnasiums with your child and exercising could be another way of bonding and developing a healthy regime for the future. Focusing on sporting skills like having a kick of the footy or a hit of cricket with your child helps encourages them to practise these skills in their play time with other children.

According to TCM Medicine the following conditions are aggravated by these foods:
- Eczema: The worst thing to give a child with eczema is beef. Beef includes hamburger mince, veal and beef sausages. It has

to be removed from the diet for a minimum of three months before seeing any improvement. (This doesn't mean all red meat. Lamb, chicken, pork and so on are fine.)

- Asthma: The worst thing to give a child with asthma is banana. Again after three months you should see improvement. Milk also falls into this category although it is not as severe as banana.

- ADHD: From my own experience anything with chilli, red food colouring and lots of sugar will send the child up the wall and also anything that contains caffeine. Although it may seem counterintuitive that you would give a child caffeine, a large number of times I've seen children as young as five wander into the clinic sucking on a cola drink from a fast-food chain, while the parents are beside themselves trying to control the child's behaviour. By simply removing all these things and cutting out the sugar, within a few weeks it is like having a completely different child come to see you. In addition to the eczema, beef also makes young children very aggressive. Naturally taking it out of the diet goes a long way to resolving the problem.

Television

Here's something else you may like to consider. I believe that part of the present problem with society becoming more over-weight revolves around television habits. There are two things in particular. The first is parents who use the TV as a babysit-ter – I believe this would have a big impact on a young child's mind and teaches the child to associate what's on TV as a primary source of entertainment. When they grow up, this association is still there at the subconscious level, so adults wanting entertainment will simply turn on the television rather than looking elsewhere. Secondly, TV entertainment has had long enough to play with the formula (over 50 years) and I believe networks have grown very sophisticated in knowing what keeps people 'glued' to the set. In the old days we used to call the TV 'the idiot box'. You never hear this said anymore and I am wondering why. Is it because as time has gone on we have become more accustomed to television in our lives or have the networks figured out what it is that we like to see? Have you ever been having a conversation in a bar or other public place when there is a TV on and noticed how people's attention seems to be drawn to what is on the set? Why does the TV have this hypnotic effect on people?

Here are some interesting points about television.

- The average person watches between four to four and a half hours of television per day.
- The average student spends more time watching television than in the classroom.
- The average television viewer sees up to 20 acts of violence per hour.
- On average, only one out of every five acts of violence on television and in movies is properly punished.
- Lifelong television viewing habits can be established by age three.
- The American Academy of Child and Adolescent Psychiatry, the American Academy of Pediatrics and the

---

American Psychological Association all agree that violence in the media is related to aggression in real life.

- On average, people see 30,000 television commercials each year.
- In households where the TV is always left on, 34 per cent of four- to 6-year-olds can read and 56 per cent can read in homes that watch less TV.
- People who watch a lot of television read less than those who don't.
- Television stories are fast-paced, giving people a distorted sense of time.
- Television commercials encourage people to crave products indiscriminately.

People who watch TV read less . . . so does that mean by you reading this book that you are an exception?

The fussy eater

A problem parents face is the child who refuses to eat what's put in front of them. There are many books devoted to how to make children eat. Games you can play, funny faces you can make, special types of meals and so on. Knowing that there is always an alternative approach to any given situation, I spoke with a number of parents who never had problems with their child's eating. I reached an unexpected conclusion. It seemed to me that the parents who didn't make a big issue about whether or not the child ate, seemed to have less trouble, if any, feeding their children. Here's my explanation.

Children need attention and are constantly exploring ways of getting it. When they find a way of getting the attention they pursue it avidly. This is why you get the good child/bad child syndrome. The good child gets the attention in the form of reward for their behaviour while the bad child gets attention by being punished. They both end up with what they want: the parent's attention. Good or bad it doesn't matter, it still gets you to the same destination. The fussy or stubborn child basically holds all the cards at meal time. They can control their parent's behaviour by simply refusing to eat – it's that easy. All they have to do is hold out for as long as possible and while this goes on, the child gets mileage from the way it's behaving. It has the parent's attention.

There was always something in the back of my mind with this situation. Having met more than my fair share of people with eating disorders, in many cases there is an underlying theme – that of control. In this context the person usually has no control over their life and has discovered that they can control people around them by controlling the lowest common denominator, what they eat. By doing this, the person regains what their life has always lacked, that of control over the people around them. We know that early childhood experiences creates patterns of behaviour that play themselves out in adult life. I believe that this may be one of them.

To understand this, I spoke to the experts, both professionals and parents themselves, who never had fussy eaters. I wanted to find out why and was surprised to discover that the strategy they found worked best was not to buy into the

245

control drama. If the child didn't eat what was on the table it just went hungry. Now before you reach for the phone and start calling the clinic in protest, just consider a couple of points. Firstly this was the strategy that a lot of people found worked. Why? Children's early education is learning about choices. Because the child learns that all that happens when it doesn't want to eat, is it goes to bed hungry. This teaches the child about choice and the consequences of those choices. It makes the child responsible for it's decisions instead of the parents. It learns that the consequence of not eating is an empty belly. Basically, the premise of the parents was 'when they are hungry they'll eat'. This is reasonable assumption and should not be confused with a parent who refuses to take responsibility for feeding their child.

The other thing that adds weight to my argument is the cases of undernourished children in Australia are 'extremely rare'. Conversely, as I described earlier, overfed children who as a result of eating food that has little or no nutrition value are often overweight and malnourished. I think the risk of the child being undernourished by letting it not eat when its not hungry is offset by the problems of creating a control drama by trying to force the child to eat. From parents I spoke with, letting the child go to bed was the easiest solution and the child soon learnt to eat when the family eats, otherwise it goes hungry. As a result they never had the problem of making the child eat. The flow-on effect is the child learns from sitting at the table and eating to mimic adult behaviour and develop social and interpersonal skills within the family.

Parents are always interested in learning more about childhood behaviour and I know I could write volumes.

Essentially, for children the goal for their behaviour is orientated to getting attention from the parents. To a child, the parent's attention is like oxygen, they can't survive without it. For some children it doesn't matter if it's a good or bad, if the child doesn't think they are getting enough then they can become desperate.

For now here is a short summary.

There are four modes of childhood behaviour/misbehaviour:

- **Getting attention**: Whether it be rewarded for good behaviour or punished for bad behaviour it's still the same. If the child believes that this isn't paying dividends then it goes on to the next mode.

- **Seizing attention**: Things like 'look at me mummy I've climbed the tree' or 'look at me mummy I'm putting "pussy" in the dryer'. If this doesn't work the child can eventually go onto the third mode.

- **Revenge**: Getting revenge against the parents for not paying enough attention by doing things that really annoys, hurts or upset them. You see this often in older children like getting tattoos or piercing or weird hairdos and so on and finally if this all fails then usually the last mode is . . .

- **Withdrawal**: The child becomes withdrawn. If your thinking little Johnny or Mary is already at this point then may be you should talk to someone about it.

If you want to learn more about childhood behaviour then a book I recommend to parents is written by Professor Maurice Balsam called *Becoming Better Parents*.

Some helpful tips:

Set a good example for your children. I cannot stress this enough. Children learn from observation. If the parents don't 'walk the walk and talk the talk' then it's hard to expect the children to do so. Practice healthy eating habits and enjoy regular physical activity together. Make it a part of your family quality time.

Don't use food as a reward or a means of shaping behaviour. Ask yourself if a child is hungry for something emotional, rather than food. Find other ways of rewarding a child. Food gives immediate gratification, which can become addictive.

Focus on health rather than weight. The most successful approaches focus on feeling better. It is better to encourage a child to see that the healthy choices they are making up are for health rather than weight loss. Children do not need an authority figure to remind them that they have a weight problem. Use your authority to encourage the child and to complement them on their progress.

Don't ban food. If you take something out of the diet, be careful not to 'appear' to ban it outright. Children become fixated on things that are 'forbidden' and may seek it out when away from home. Banning things also allows people indirectly associated with your children to score points, like grandparents giving them the things that they are not allowed. Better to have some sort of strategy that still allows the child to have certain things at appropriate times, with the understanding of where they fit into the diet. Remember, be an educator. Education builds motivation.

Take charge. Don't turn over food decisions to kids. It's the parents' responsibility to provide healthy meals; it's the child's decision whether or not to eat.

Turn off the television. Twenty per cent of children's food intake is done in front of television. Not surprisingly a lot of the food the children want to eat at this time is the same food that is advertised during the children's program. Parents may be unaware of the various ads children watch – food companies are very clever and know their target audience. Fast-food companies often advertise during children's favourite shows. They know that if they don't get them while they are young, then they will not grow up as adults depending on their food. Limit TV time to less than two hours a day. Instead of TV and video games, encourage your child to play active games or participate in sports for fun.

Don't fill the child up with drinks before the meal. Many parents give the children various drinks that make the child feel full before it sits down to eat – as a result they are not hungry.

Avoid quick fixes. Being 'on a diet' may be an effective way to lose weight but you have to avoid the on-again off-again syndrome with children – it does nothing for their self-esteem. Aim for permanent changes in food intake – gradual weight loss should be the goal. Praise and encourage your child as they start to lose the weight, compliment them on how well they look. Try to monitor their progress beyond weighing them. Feeling good, more energy and looser clothing are all good indicators of progress. The simple fact that the child is losing weight gradually is enough, it is important not to make an issue of the child's weight, so use the scales sparingly. A child is growing rapidly, physically and mentally, and a healthy diet is important at this time. Weight loss may not be reflected on the scales simply because they are getting bigger, especially with boys.

Don't overfeed. Forcing the child to eat makes them override their own feelings of being full. Introduce new things slowly and gradually. If they are not hungry then don't panic, they will eat anything put in front of them if they are hungry enough.

Never say diet. It's all about health and happiness and the right choices and above all your love for them.

CHAPTER 6

I've lost the weight, now what?

Before we go any further, you need to ask yourself should I be reading this? If you haven't started following the book already, then there is no point in reading this next section. However, if you have now reached your desired weight and achieved what you have set out to do, then by all means continue.

What you are now trying to achieve is a balance between what you have learned and the way you used to eat before. Bear in mind that your old habits were the cause of the weight and other health problems in the first place, so the more you gravitate towards that style of eating the more the problems will return. This would be an undesirable outcome, considering the progress you have made already. As with most people when they reach this stage, they are tempted to reward themselves with eating bad carbs. You're in for a surprise as you soon discover what comes from bombarding your body with sugar and bad carbs again. Once you have gotten this out of your system the next process is about tailoring what you learned to suit your lifestyle.

Up until now, keeping the blood sugar levels under control and stopping the liver from storing glycogen has been one of the keys to your success. Now that you are no longer trying to lose weight, raising your blood sugar levels and keeping glycogen from the liver is not such a big issue, however what does become important now is the amount of fat included in your diet.

Here's what happens. Up until now you've been eating two types of meals, the moderate carbohydrate and the protein meals. Now you can start mixing the two menus together. This means having rice with fish, meat sauce on your pasta with parmesan cheese, butter on the toast, milk in your tea and so on, however when you do this you have to keep the fats down to a minimum. The reason, of course, is because the moderate carbs will still elicit insulin and whatever fats are included will be absorbed – nothing has changed. So basically you are using the moderate GI carbs and low GI carbs together while adding protein to the meal. It is best to leave the high GI foods out of the picture wherever possible. If you eat something that is high GI once in awhile, it's probably not going to be a big issue, however if you continue eating high GI foods then you may as well forget about all the good work you have done – you will find the weight will just start creeping back on but what really becomes an issue at this stage is the fat in the diet. Because you are now exposing yourself to the effects of insulin, then you have to start policing the fat once again. For many people not eating fat is exactly what they did originally with varying results. If this prospect doesn't thrill you, then you're not alone and you may prefer an alternate approach.

The other choice is to follow the book, exactly as you have been doing before, but have the occasional meal that falls outside of the guidelines once in a while. When you have one of these meals you are still being mindful of not eating high-fat things, but you are not worrying so much because most of the time you have been doing everything by the book. Going out to dinner with friends and so on is not such a big problem because whatever damage you did should be compensated for the rest of the time you have been eating correctly.

Most people follow the book through the week and tend to relax on the weekends. This approach can allow you to lose whatever you may have put on during the weekend, assuming you don't binge. From experience most people will experiment and find what best suits them. In practical terms they usually end up with something like this. You will find in the long run you will most likely fall into the pattern of eating low GI most of the time. Most people prefer this way of eating and for good reason – low GI meals are tasty, filling, make you feel good and you don't put on weight so why not just keep using the knowledge? If, for social reasons, you sit down and eat and drink whatever, if this is every so often, with a bit of luck, you should find that your weight should stay pretty much the same. However if you overdo the entertaining and you find that the weight is starting to creep back again, then it's a simple matter of going back to doing everything 'strictly by the book' for a few weeks to lose the extra kilos. Be careful though, it is very easy to get out of control and you need to have a very conservative approach to these social outings.

Alcohol

Drinking alcohol, as we all know, is a social lubricant and if we drink in moderation then there are plenty of health benefits, however if you find that you're getting 'lubricated' a little bit too often, you will find that looking after your weight can also become a problem. Getting drunk tends to diminish responsibility and lowers inhibition and it is very easy to start off with the best intentions only to find the next morning you have completely made a dog's breakfast of it all. Drinking alcohol and eating a high-fat food is not such a good idea because all that happens is the fat in the meal gets absorbed. If I am going to drink alcohol or anything else that is going to raise my blood sugar levels, I am always mindful that the fat in the food is going to be absorbed, so I always make an effort to keep fat to a minimum. What I find a lot easier is to have control over when I decide to drink. When I am at home for example and planning on enjoying a bottle of red, I will always be sure to have a moderate carbohydrate meal. Why? Because a moderate carbohydrate meal is also a low-fat meal, this way you can enjoy the wine without the worry.

If you include alcohol with your meal, then my advice is be careful not to drink alcohol with high-fat foods, wherever possible. Avoiding fats whilst drinking alcohol is a proven approach. Lowering inhibitions makes it difficult to eat healthily and not to fall in a heap. By keeping the rules simple, it allows for a greater chance of success. If you like to drink then

I suggest you follow this formula. I think for the most part this is why people associate alcohol with putting on weight.

There once was a very successful system of controlling the weight here in Australia called 'Gut Busters'. The principles were very simple and aimed at men who had developed a 'beer gut'. They just told the men that if they drank alcohol, it had to be in moderation and they must not eat fattening things.

In addition, the total amount of fat they could consume in a day had to be no more than 35 grams. The men had a little pocketbook, which listed the amount of fat in every type of food, so they simply limited the fat in the diet and made sure that when they drank they did it in moderation and avoided eating fattening things. This worked for a lot of people and thousands of men in Australia were able to lose the beer gut. What happened next may surprise you; an American weight loss company bought them out and shut them down to get rid of competition.

What 'Gut Busters' had discovered was when people drink they tended to gravitate towards fattening things. By simply avoiding things like beer nuts, takeaway, fried foods and so on, they were able to get rid of the expanded waistline.

While still on the subject, as we all know, there are a great many varieties of alcohol to choose from and it seems that everyone has a favourite. Unfortunately if your favourite is the kind that is high in sugar and carbohydrate, then life can be difficult if you are trying to maintain your weight. When alcohol is made, the sugar from the carbohydrates is converted into alcohol. Alcohol generally is low in carbohydrate, it's usually what they are mixed with that contains the sugar. Think carefully about what you are planning to use, as most are little more than high sugar soft drinks. A can of rum and cola for example, is just a sugar bombshell because of the cola. You may have to consider some of the diet soft drinks as an alternative in your spirit.

Testing the GI of alcohol has not met with a great deal of success over the years and unfortunately there is very little reference material. The main problem is the process of having a group of volunteers sitting down and drinking straight spirits for a while and then expecting them to wait patiently for a few hours while they get the blood sugar levels tested usually fails. Most of them have either passed out, are trying to 'pash' each other or have already left the building in search of a lamb souvlaki or curry vindaloo.

Scotch whisky is one spirit that reportedly has a zero GI. Unfortunately for other spirits we can only go by the amount of carbohydrates and calories. Vodka, rum and bourbon have similar values when compared to Scotch. So theoretically drinking these either straight up or with soda or diet mixer should be okay. Not having tried it myself I cannot vouch for any of it. A number of patients have tried mixing Scotch whisky and diet cola together and reportedly they drank this concoction after their protein meals and carb meals without any ill effects. I myself have never felt the need and I wouldn't recommend mixing it with the protein meal, for the obvious reasons that the sweetness in the diet cola would be enough to get an insulin response, but I feel that it is worth mentioning in the maintenance phase, as it may be applicable to you.

So if you don't drink spirits, then what is left is beer and wine. I have read various articles about how the amount of carbohydrates in the beer is similar to wine and this may be true. Like I said, if you were able to drink beer in moderation, you may find that your weight will remain the same, however most Australian men have no idea what drinking beer in moderation actually is. (24 beers in a slab, 24 hours in a day . . . coincidence?) I have read the information about carbohydrate in beer and on paper it's comparable to wine, so in this context, I have no explanation as to why beer seems to make people put on weight so much. I have always avoided drinking beer whenever possible as I find it is a sure way to start putting on weight, but you can be your own judge on this one.

You may find when trying to look after your weight, alcohol is an Achilles heel. Lowering inhibitions and diminishing responsibility on one hand makes it difficult to be selective about what you are eating on the other. Alcohol also dilates the blood vessels in the stomach and your digestion really starts to wind up in preparation for food, so it is best to plan ahead if you find yourself in this situation and think about some moderate carb meals to go with your food.

For many years we have advised people on the maintenance phase that wine is the best choice. Wine is something that has many great health benefits, and there are numerous articles that have been written on the effects of drinking wine in moderation. Wine is rich in antioxidants, something that protects you from ageing, and because it is a vasodilator it is also good for preventing heart attack. When making the choice between white or red, red has more of these properties and is lower in carbohydrate as well. Another feature about red wine is it's very high in iron. Choose red over white when possible.

Think about what you have learnt so far. You have discovered how controlling your blood sugar levels makes an incredible difference to your weight and, as you can appreciate, you have had to be very careful about what you were eating to achieve that. Unless you continue to use your judgment correctly, being able to eat rich foods and not put on weight will not work for you at all. The protection that this book has offered you up until now will become non-existent once you've crossed the line.

When you have a high carb meal, the glycogen returns to the liver once more. As a result it takes three days before the body is back in a state for the weight to come off again. So for arguments sake, you follow the book six days a week, and have one meal on the seventh day that includes bad carbs, it will take another three days for your body to go back to normal, then for a few more days the weight will start coming down before the seventh day when you repeat the process again. Throw in another meal here and there and one can see how easy it is to not be receiving much benefit from the GI. You must try to be sensible.

Festive seasons

The festive season, birthdays and the occasional get-together can usually be a time of extended and eating and drinking. I find that during this time it becomes increasingly difficult to maintain a healthy eating pattern. The best strategy is to minimise the exposure to the high fat and high sugar intake, meaning when you are able to eat low GI as per the book, do so. Don't make the excuse that because you ate something that you 'shouldn't have' the day before, then you may as well do the same the next day. What will happen is you can easily get out of control, and soon find that your weight will start to come back on again.

For me, Christmas and New Year is about catching up with friends, going out, having a good time. But the days in between I always eat low GI like it's my last meal on earth. What I am trying to do is stop my weight getting ridiculous. Like most people I hate being overweight, and if I hadn't been looking for some solution back in 1995, then I would never have discovered the glycemic index. Usually, after New Year, things settle down and return to normal and it will be in the intervening months before Easter that I will vigorously follow low GI losing the extra kilos that I inevitably put on over Christmas and New Year. Easter is the last milestone in the 'bad eating calendar', before you can settle into a nice comfortable routine. It always comes as a surprise during these episodes where you realise how much you enjoy following a low GI diet. There is no doubt that a few hours after the Christmas lunch you are normally feeling very unwell and wondering why you ate too much, not to mention wearing a stupid paper hat. This is a good opportunity to reflect back on your choices prior to this, and realise the many benefits you have enjoyed from understanding the glycemic index.

Food rewards

For one who has been following the GI for more than a decade, episodes of interrupting your pattern of eating, like Christmas and birthdays, dinner with friends and so on, are predictable, and initially in the early years, I admit, I looked forward to having a break from the routine. We are creatures of habit after all, who enjoy doing things differently from time to time. In the early days I truly believed that times when the meal wasn't low GI it was some kind of treat. Many people who are experiencing the GI for the first time will often see things this way. However as time went by, I was surprised to discover that I started to resist these moments more and more, simply because I was enjoying the pleasures of eating low GI. I will give you an example.

My mother lives in the UK. She visits Australia once a year. The food in the UK, historically, is quite awful, and although my mother is German, she has grown very fond of Chinese food from living in Australia. Of course there is no Chinese food in the UK of any great quality that compares to the variety here. Consequently when she arrives, the first thing she likes to do is visit her favourite Chinese restaurants, with Chérie under one arm and me under another. Unfortunately there is nothing low GI about Chinese food. Each year that Mum would visit I would look forward to this. I'm not complaining, having been involved in Chinese medicine my entire adult life I, like my Mum, was fond of Chinese food. Unfortunately by the time Mum was climbing aboard the plane we had both put on a number of kilos in the process. It came as a surprise to discover that even Mum's annual visits started to concern me. Deep down I really wish I could follow the way I had come to enjoy during the rest of the year. It came as a great relief one year, when my mother had complained about her weight, that I finally convinced her to read my book.

It may seem odd that she hadn't already but when it comes to your immediate family, it is not a given that they will take your advice no matter how qualified it is. After my mother read the book, she not only understood it, she became passionate about it. She lost around about nine kilos, about one stone, and became an advocate of the low GI to all her friends. I personally think it is very good that an elderly woman can apply this knowledge and lose a considerable amount of weight in the process.

Last year when Mum visited us the Chinese restaurants were thankfully not on the agenda – instead we cooked for her and, with the exception of the occasional bottle of wine and an eightieth birthday cake, she followed the principles of the book to the letter.

Colder weather

Something else that you should also be aware of is the effects of winter. As I write, I am sitting in Melbourne, Australia and as luck would have it, it's winter. If you live in a part of the world that's warm most of the time, then more power to you. The cold may not affect you, but if you are just like me, then the cold becomes an issue when it comes to weight loss. Your body prefers to put on weight during the colder months, so you may find that the weight can be a little more stubborn than at other times of the year. Always remember the old adage. 'If you want to be slim in summer, keep the weight off in winter'. This is exactly right. So resist the temptation to start putting weight on during winter because there will be a natural tendency for your body to do so. I normally allow myself a couple of kilos for insulation, but if you 'fall asleep at the wheel', you will find that when the weather gets warmer and you begin to peel the layers of clothing away, don't be surprised if you are not as slim as before. Conversely if you are trying to lose weight during the winter months, assuming you actually have a winter, you may find you are not losing it quite as quickly as you may have wished. Don't let this deter you because you will find as the weather gets warmer the rate at which you lose the weight will increase along with the mercury. As the years go by and the more experienced you become, the better you will be at keeping your weight stable during winter, and the better the results will be in the long run.

So what are you to do now? Here are the main principles again. Once you have the hang of it, it becomes second nature.

1. Stick with following low GI, as set down in this book as much as possible.
2. Don't overcompensate when you go out for a meal, and stuff yourself with bad carbs.
3. If you're drinking alcohol, then drink wine, preferably red. Avoid beer.
4. When having alcohol, make sure to keep fat to a minimum. Have it with a carb meal is the best bet.
5. Try to keep the high/bad carb meals (if any) confined to the weekend, followed by the longest possible number of days of low GI food.
6. Keep an eye on your weight during winter and don't let it get out of hand.

You may find that some of these principles are more important to you then others. Don't be surprised if you make up a few of your own. One way or another, you will eventually arrive at a comfortable fit with this knowledge. Even though understanding the basics and achieving your goals can be quite easy, it may take a number of years before you can really say that you have this whole thing down pat. Like many people, when you look back you know that there is no possibility of eating the way you did before without going back to square one, but it may take you a few years before you realise this. Save yourself the trouble and just stick with what you have learnt. Using the GI is quite brilliant and many concerns that you may have had about your health and your weight has all but vanished.

Conclusion

This knowledge is now yours to keep. Give yourself time to become accustomed to it and just like every beginner there will always be a teething process. If you make a mistake don't worry, just keep going. As time goes by you will get better and more used to making the necessary choices about your food.

What happens from here on out is all up to you. Remember that no one can take better care of you than yourself. Being able to control your weight and taking care of your health should be easier than ever before. You are now part of an exclusive club.

As you become more accustomed to using the GI and the information in this book, you will become more and more aware of what you have learned. For a very small investment you now have something that can potentially change your life forever.

I hope that reading this has taught you more about yourself and the relationship with what you eat.

Good luck for the future.

Yours in good health.

John Ratcliffe Dip TCM, Grad Dip Psy

Appendices

Just a brief note to explain that a frequent comment made by readers was they wished I would talk in more depth about some of the issues I touch upon. So I have made an attempt to flesh out a few topics that I felt may be of further interest and although it is not critical to understand these things, it may help broaden your knowledge base for greater success.

Please note: I have tried to avoid the boring diatribe but I can't guarantee the risk of an unexpected attack of narcolepsy.

Appendix A: The psychology of eating

Ancient survival mechanisms meets modern day

Society is changing dramatically. Over the past 100 years we've seen the advent of modern medicine and the industrial revolution. In the past 50 we've seen space flight, television and computers. The last 20 years has seen changes in communications, the Internet and the mapping of the human genome. We are moving so fast that some analysts expect that by the year 2050 the technology curve will start to go straight up. As far as progress with our bodies is concerned, other than a thinner skull and less hair, nothing has really changed for a few hundred THOUSAND years. Just think about it for a moment – it's not like we originally had lungs in our buttocks and feet on backwards and eventually we developed technology and changed the way we are. The physiology of the body is something that has changed very slowly over time. Our bodies have taken a very long time to develop and above all there is one function that the body excels at, that of survival. For the body to survive it needs energy and when it comes to absorbing energy, the body is very, very good at it.

You may wonder where I am going with all this, but it is important to bear in mind that our bodies are about survival. Western medicine is beginning to discover what the Chinese had learnt many thousands of years ago. The body is extremely sophisticated and it has many mechanisms for coping with a variety of situations – in fact it is so good that it allows us to get away with murder. Let me give you an example.

For argument's sake, lets say that the penalty for overeating was fits and seizures, then no one would overeat. If the penalty for smoking a cigarette was blindness, then no one would smoke and so on. The fact is our body can cope with all sorts of things, and because it does, we conclude that it must be all right to do so. Many reasons why the body is able to do these things are firmly rooted in our past. Living in an urban environment has only occurred in the past few hundred years, and as we look further back along our evolutionary trail, our origins began as hunter-gathers. Life was very different then when getting regular food was hardly reliable. Our bodies developed ways of coping with these obstacles and these are same mechanisms that we live with, day-to-day in our present age. Starvation diets, for example, cause the body to hold on to the fat and burn muscle, an ancient survival mechanism.

Asthma is a common problem, especially here in Australia. Asthma is an autoimmune response that occurs when the lung comes in contact with dust, pollen and so on. It is believed that asthma is actually an ancient autoimmune response there to protect us from parasites. The lung thinks that dust and pollen is actually attacking its surface and responds by creating inflammation at the site to destroy the problem and uses mucus to flush it away. Of course nowadays we are not threatened with inhaling parasites, beyond dust mites, which we have other means of dealing with. A vacuum cleaner would be a good example. Unfortunately for the asthma sufferer, when this autoimmune response kicks in, they become short of breath, find it difficult to breathe and usually need Ventolin to counteract the response.

Stress can be seen as another example of an ancient mechanism functioning in modern day. In the good old days, when we were out in the jungle gathering food, the dangers we faced were quite tangible, whether it be attack by an animal or falling off something or being drowned in a river. The answer was quite simple — we avoided the situation or just ran away from it. Stress and anxiety is a signal to the body that we are in danger. Normally when placed in this situation our instinct is to take flight and run away, thereby reducing stress and returning things to normal. Unfortunately for us, when threatened by a stressful situation we can't simply take off. If that were the case we would spend a great part of our days running and hiding from just about everything. What we do instead is the exact opposite. We resist the instinct, and stay and subject ourselves to this perceived danger. This conflict of interest causes great strain on our central nervous system. On one hand we consciously recognise that it would be inappropriate whenever a problem arises to just run away. On the other hand there is a part of us subconsciously telling us we need to escape. As a result it stresses the individual as they try to resolve the difference between what their head is telling them and their feelings. That's why stress is perceptional, and some people can cope better than others and why changing the way we think about certain things will change the way we experience them.

Brain Chemistry

So back to the subject at hand. Another unique feature is our take on food. Remember, the body's primary function is to survive and to do this, it requires energy, and energy comes from food. That food is always carbohydrate, and it's no surprise that the body will always choose the carbohydrates with the most energy. Again for argument's sake, let's say that you are standing in the Savannah of Africa and it's 300,000 years BC. You have been eating grass to survive, and you discover honey for the first time. Do you take a taste of it, think 'hmmmm okay', and then go back to eating the grass again? Of course not, your brain would tell you to start to eat the honey (we can ignore the fact that you are probably getting stung by now). So why did you choose to eat the honey in the first place – how did you know it was better than eating grass? Your brain had to tell you and to do this it uses chemicals, which affect the way you feel about what you are eating. These chemicals influence your desire to continue eating more. The thing is we continue to experience this in the present day. On one level we believe that we make our food choices consciously, however there are very sophisticated mechanisms at play that in fact make these choices for you. If we were to look back over history we would see that when a certain food becomes available, they grow in popularity because of their flavour and taste. For example, when millers discovered a way of grinding flour to an almost talcum-like perfection it became the toast of Europe, no pun intended.

If we take it one step further and combine the high energy food with fats, then our brain chemistry is in heaven. We've got the combination right and by providing two sources of high energy food we are rewarded with a nice feeling. Of course feeling sick and bloated an hour or so later is beside the point. We have achieved our primary objective of absorbing the food in the first place and we move on. The way that we deal with food revolves very heavily around our body's primary function of survival. And if we were to examine the food we have included in a day-to-day life it's no coincidence that our 'favourite' foods are always the combination of fats and carbohydrates.

Going back to the example I made earlier, about deciding what to eat 300,000 years ago. If you had a choice between eating roots, leaves, grass, dung and bugs or takeaway what would you choose? As our society has evolved, we have gradually added to the menu more and more of our 'favourite' foods, so much so, that the choices have become the same and as I have pointed out earlier, the effect on our health has been devastating. Every so often I might catch a cooking show and watch a chef prepare a delicious meal. I sit in fascination when the meal takes on the appearance of being low GI. I know inevitably at some point he will add something that has a high GI. I'm always interested to know at what point does it come in. Will it be in the beginning with one of the basic ingredients or will come in the middle or at the end? Without fail something will appear that raises the blood sugar levels and allows whatever fat is in the meal to be absorbed. Without it the meal becomes meaningless to the body. What is the point of putting all that food on the plate without being able to absorb the energy. As you and I both know, without the high GI carbs we can still enjoy the meal and instead of gaining weight we can lose it.

The fact is the risk of starvation in a modern-day society is as unlikely as being trampled by wild poodles, but as far as the body is concerned starvation is waiting behind every corner and any moment the food will run out and famine commence. Of course I'm not saying that can never happen, but you get the picture (poodles have been known to run in gangs). The thing is, even though we can wax, shape, suck, colour and change their appearance, our bodies are still living relics of the past. Our relationship with survival has quite cleverly manipulated our choices of cuisine to favour the best possible combinations to get what the body wants most, high-energy food. So what are we to do?

In modern-day society we have to practise modern thinking. Of course we can have eyes bigger than our stomachs when surrounded by food. In spite of this we have to make the correct choices for our health and longevity. In the same way that we have to do exercise to compensate for the fact that we are no longer as active as yesteryear, we must exercise our ability to make the correct choices of what to eat. For many people low GI has been the most suitable. The fact that living in today's society we can eat whatever we like whenever we like is of little consequence. Simply because it's there isn't good enough. When your body and those 'pleasure' chemicals start telling you to eat something that's really not going to be doing you any good, you can ignore it if you want. It not really 'you' who wants it but rather your body and its weird survival agenda. How many times have you sat and wondered, 'What the hell was I thinking' or 'I know I shouldn't be eating this'? Just stop and think about it and see if you can separate yourself from what you are feeling and what you are thinking and let your thinking lead for a change. Nothing terrible will happen and you will go on to live another day, trust me. Being indifferent to these urges is something that you will become more familiar with as time goes by. Often people comment that they are amazed to discover that their food cravings have vanished. This is because those wild and crazy chemicals are no longer firing off inside their brain. It can also come as a shock when they're reintroduced to the menu, that the cravings returned like new.

Emerging epidemic of preventable illness

Like most people, I had become acutely aware that we are facing an overweight epidemic. While trying to get a handle on the situation, I have looked at numerous reports on why the Western world and in particular Australians are getting fatter. It seems like society needs someone to blame. Fast-food companies have been taken to court for making people fat, children's advertising on television has been blamed, even the parents for raising lazy children and being overprotective, have all come under severe scrutiny. Even the WHO has criticised the sugar industry, which is an enormous departure from their standard and ineffectual advice of eat less fat. So while we are staring into our collective navels trying to generate some kind of idea of the problem, I have my own opinion. History and evolution provides great insight into the physiology of the body but is not sufficient enough to explain why we should all of a sudden find ourselves in the past 20 years with this burgeoning health problem. There are a couple more pieces to the puzzle that deserve a mention.

Australians are working longer hours than ever before. Believe it or not, Australia is almost the hardest-working country in the world. There is only one other country where people work similar hours, and that country is South Korea. Could you possibly imagine that Australia and South Korea

272

have had something like that in common? Unfortunately for many people, just getting ahead has become an intense struggle. At the time of writing this book, I had just stopped working seven days a week to working five days, for the first time in three-and-a-half years. Unfortunately for Chérie, she is still going at it. When I read this report, I had little trouble understanding how Australians are the hardest-working people in the world. I live in the city and nearly all of my patients work and they all seem to be in the same boat, some more than others. Women are having their children later in life. It's very common for women in their thirties to just be starting a family. It has taken them this long to see the financial security needed to start a family. So why has it becomes so hard to get ahead? You may also be surprised to learn that Australia is the fourth-highest taxed country in the world – the French have the honour of being the highest. For example, to go into the highest taxed bracket of 49 cents in the dollar, one needs to earn over $60,000 per year. By contrast, in US, to go into the same tax bracket, one needs to be earning $550,000 per year. So what does all this mean? It is quite simple, to get anywhere in Australia you need to work harder than ever before. People are working longer hours, starting families later, there is higher household debt, and most families have a double income. Quality of life is going down the proverbial. Looking at it from this perspective it is easy to understand why people find looking after their health and eating right a very low priority. As a result they are making very poor food choices and suffering the inevitable consequences.

The other problem is that technology has provided us with instant gratification. For example if I want to talk to someone, I can use a mobile phone to call their mobile and speak to them instantly. I can use the same phone to get the latest news, weather or sports scores any time of the day. If that's not entertaining enough, I can SMS my friends absurd messages if I get bored and, while on the subject of entertainment, should it be my desire I can watch movies in cinema-like quality on my plasma screen TV (that is of course if I had the money to buy one), with surround sound and digital pictures beamed in via satellite, with 80 channels to choose from. I could watch the war in Iraq, learn about the whales, watch a swimsuit competition and watch a walk in space all by the press a button. If I get hungry, I have an endless variety of takeaway menus to choose from. I can make a phone call and piping hot food will be delivered to my door shortly thereafter. When driving my car, I can get traffic reports, information about weather, outside temperature, fuel economy, I can even get a little voice telling me how far ahead the next turn is, and also when I have arrived. If I turn on the CD player, I have hours of my favourite artists to listen to. If I think I'm getting a little over stimulated, it's time to make my online holiday reservations and look forward to doing nothing on some island, to unwind. The point is we have become used to the idea of things happening in a hurry. Unfortunately food slips very neatly into the category of instant gratification. When we 'feel the urge', all you need to do is pay your money, open your mouth and pop it in. Immediately you get a terrific taste and the smell and sensation overwhelm you. Your brain chemistry starts to fire up, and guess what? You're feeling better already. This is a trap.

When we have an itch that needs to be scratched, we don't wait. Even as I sit here typing, (as I mentioned, rugged up against the bitter Melbourne cold, too stingy to turn on the

274

heater) my computer is linked to the Internet 24 hours a day. Via high speed connection, I can pull up instant information at my frozen fingertips. If I want to find something out about what's happening, with say a certain pharmaceutical company, I can type in to my Google search engine and find out straight away. It even tells me, in hundredths of a second, how long it took to find the answer.

Let's face it, life is all about choice, and if there is one thing in life that it all should know it is 'We must be responsible for our choices, and live by the choices that we make'. My mission has been to empower the individual, to take charge of their health and make the right and informed choices, and the food that we eat plays a major role in our health. But responsibility does not rest squarely on the shoulders of the individual. The fact is it's a social problem as well. So when patients are struggling with their food cravings, I encourage them to try to think of it in different ways.

Knowing that it is simply instant gratification that you seek, one can think of preparing low GI food as a way of putting off the gratification until later and thereby enjoying it all the more.

So there are four pieces to the puzzle to take into account when considering health and eating.

1. Our bodies have a predisposition to absorbing energy and, when allowed to, will keep absorbing energy *ad infinititum*. So it's important not to provide it an opportunity is to absorb energy it doesn't need.
2. There is high-energy food all around us and whether it be because of clever marketing for social conditioning, it is

irrelevant to a person following low GI. We must exercise the correct choice in what to eat.

3. We all work very hard and time is a precious commodity. We have to have clear strategies on how to provide the appropriate food for ourselves. If this means using some of that precious time to prepare food in advance and enjoying the process of preparing the food, so be it.

4. We have a tendency to want instant gratification; with it comes compulsive behaviour. Finding other ways to meet these various demands beyond food needs to be explored. Relaxing to music, having a bath, relaxing in a spa, watching a movie, holding hands, getting a cuddle or thinking about the sense of achievement that comes with reaching your goals. All can move you away from being in the moment.

We should take a moment to appreciate the food that we eat. For example, it wasn't that long ago when families used to say grace at the table. We no longer seem to appreciate the fact that simply having something to eat is a blessing.

Everyday I am reminded of the enjoyment and benefits I have gained from following the glycemic index. If I ever wonder what life would have been like without it, I only need to look to my old friends to have an idea of what yours truly would be like had he not discovered the GI in time. It ain't pretty!

As the final thought, consider the types of food that we find on offer to us each day. Take a moment to reflect and ask yourself, 'Would life be any better or worse today if some of these things had never been invented' and if so which ones would they be?

Appendix B: Notes for the advanced user

When reading this book, you will have realised that it has been written with the beginner in mind. However I am acutely aware that there are many people reading the book who are quite familiar with the formula and the processes and are already enjoying the experience of following my earlier works. So I would like to share with you a few thought that may help you with where you are at now.

Friends and loved ones

One unique quality of the book was the way for many years it would be passed from one person to another. Frequently a person who had read the book and had great results would come back repeatedly to the clinic to pick up more books for friends and loved ones. Being able to help other people around you is great but be aware that you also need to let people be responsible for their own choices and some people, for whatever reason, are not prepared to make the same commitment that you have. If you seem unable to motivate someone, this is not your fault. I have seen many people over the years who could really benefit from following the book but for one reason or another are unable to break away from where they are at the time. When I motivate people I do it very sparingly, because I prefer instead to be an educator. Education will always do better than motivation. The more a person understands what they are doing and why they are doing it then the motivation will come automatically.

From my experience, there can be three types of people. The first type of person reads the book, understands it, becomes extremely excited by it, follows it to the letter, loses all the weight and completely changes their life forever. The second type reads the book, loses weight, thinks 'that's all there is to it' and then slowly starts reintroducing the bad carbs into the diet. This can go one of two ways. Some people can maintain their weight this way for extended periods going back to being strict again when they overdo it. The only problem with this is there can be an incremental increase in weight and the person can find they are slowly putting the weight back on again.

I see people experimenting with what they have learnt and I believe this can be a good thing and I even encourage people to do it, once they have accomplished the initial objective. This is a part of getting good at using the information and owning the knowledge, but not everyone is going to be successful and some can get into difficulty. The solution is simple, just go back to what you where doing before and you will get the same results.

The third type of person takes your advice, reads the book and then does nothing and no amount of encouragement seems to make any difference. There can be many reasons for this behaviour; denial, control, fear, resentment to name a few. If you are to try to motivate someone close to you and you find yourself in this situation, I think it is better not to push the person but rather adopt a 'wait and see' approach. Just encouraging the person to read the book is the first step. Occasionally a patient will come to my office because their mother or daughter or someone close to them wants them to come and talk to me. Sometimes this can be a very worthwhile experience but sometimes it makes no difference at all. The person is highly resistant. I find this more in the case of teenagers for example. In this situation I don't try to convince the person that they should change their eating habits, I just encourage the person to read the book, which is fairly easy to read, and then ask them to give it a try for a week or so to see how it goes. If the person does this, I know what will happen is that they can drop a few kilos all of a sudden. This can be extremely exciting, because it comes off very easily. Now 'seize the moment' and start to encourage and motivate them to try for another week or so. If this works, you can find the person will gain momentum and make big inroads. If on the other hand, after reading the book the person is still very resistant, again don't worry. There are many complex issues that may be behind this and of course people make their own choices. It's a free country! What you may find, again from my experience, is a very unusual thing happens. The knowledge that person has gained from reading the book cannot be erased or unlearnt and even though the person chooses not to follow the advice, slowly over many months people can sometimes begin to apply little bits of what they have learnt and gradually the momentum begins. Sometimes it's important to let people just do it in their own way and in their own time. Sometimes it works, sometimes it doesn't but it is not up to you to be responsible for the choices that other people make, and you have to respect that. Often people will come to me imploring me that they can't understand why their child or husband or loved one refuses to take the plunge and get the same results. Like I said, there are complex reasons behind this and it is sometimes better to lead by example and let those around you make their decisions based on the way you are going. Beyond that it is out of your control.

The flipside to trying to motivate friends and loved ones is that they can use the same psychology on you, but in reverse! They will set bad examples in an attempt to undermine what you are doing and try to bring your progress to a halt. This is perfectly normal and predictable behaviour because what you have here is a control issue. It is best not to get into a control struggle, but simply focus on what you are doing, enjoying all the benefits from your choices and at the same time reminding those around you of the great feeling you're getting. Don't give in to temptation and be mindful of some of the traps people can set for you – that's all part of the mad games people play when they are trying undermine your best efforts. In these situations it is best to focus on yourself and redouble your efforts. It's about you, not other people. There will always be people who will be there for you and support you in your choices. You will have to work out for yourself why there are others who want to upset your progress. Don't give in to temptation – gradually over time you will win. One of the best things I did when faced with the same problem was simply say to myself 'I am just going to do today exactly what I did yesterday', and not worry about tomorrow. I just took it one day at a time until I had the momentum that just kept me going in spite of the bumps and hurdles. Perhaps you can develop your own personal motivation and sayings that help you from time to time.

Yo-yoing

From experience, occasionally a person could fluctuate between following the book and doing their own thing. Usually what happens is the weight starts to creep back, and the person gets a shock when they discover all the weight that they lost originally has returned. When people come to see me, they always feel that they have in some way failed. I never see it this way. To me it's all about learning and if someone is in the process of gradually undoing years and years of bad eating, it's sometimes unrealistic to think all they need to do is read the book and that there won't be any hiccups along the way. This person has gained a valuable insight and that cannot be undone. The person needs to reassure themselves that the old pattern of behaviour just gives the same results time and time again, overweight and unhappy. It is not unusual for people to take years before they finally have control and have turned their lives around. So give yourself time.

Cognitive styles

Even though the mechanics of the GI are very easy to understand and apply, and people can become extremely accomplished at losing and controlling their weight, there may be other factors at work. These can include emotional issues, thinking styles, social pressure and behavioural disorders, which can be extremely complex and beyond the scope of this book. Having said that, the way we think about things is the way that we will experience them. Something you learn with cognitive behavioural therapy is that the past is behind you and no amount of trying can actually erase it. Instead we learned to stop thinking about the past and instead focus on the future. The future has yet to happen and by controlling what we think about today influences what happens in the future. So cognitive behavioural therapy (CBT) focuses very much on your style of thinking and how this influences behaviour and the future. I'll give you an example.

It is not unusual for a person to come and see me who has lost a considerable amount of weight – this can sometimes be in the 40 kilo (80 pounds) and over category. Often the person is completely unprepared for the experience of being slim and the way people relate to them is totally different to before. Especially in the case of a young person, sometimes I have to have a fatherly chat explaining how to deal with the attention, but often people can become anxious that they may return to the way they once were. In this situation I ask the person to look back over their life but tell themselves that the new version of them has been the same version all along and that all through their lives they have always been very health-conscious and careful about what they eat. Now both the patient and I know that this is untrue and just fantasy, however the funny thing is the subconscious doesn't separate fantasy from reality, and if this is what you are telling it, then it has no choice but to accept it as truth. The reason why I encourage the person to think in this way is simply so the subconscious will not try to return them to their original pattern of behaviour, but instead support the new pattern and belief. I know this from experience and also from studying clinical hypnosis and cognitive behavioural therapy. If you find yourself in a similar position then I encourage you to adopt the same approach and whenever you feel anxious about where you are headed, just remind yourself that you have always been like this and have always been comfortable with the way you are. Again you may develop your own beliefs that are useful with where you are in your life and this example is one of many that may work for you.

Something quite interesting about CBT is that it's solution-orientated and focuses on the future. Here is another helpful exercise that you may wish to try. Think of the future in the way you would like to be. Sit back, relax and use your imagination. Everything had turned out to way you wanted it, you are very happy and everything is great. What would be different about you? What would have changed? What would you be doing different?

When you ask yourself these questions, make a note of the first three things you become aware of because these are the three most important things associated with your happiness and success and are, of course, the things that you should be concentrating on in your life. Sounds pretty simple I know, but the way the mind works is almost child-like in its simplicity and actually it is really that easy. I'll try to explain a little bit more.

To be or not to be, that is the question. Your subconscious works upon your beliefs and finds ways of making them become reality – it does not care if it is good or bad, it relies on you to make that distinction. It is very important that you have a good idea how you would like things to be rather than the way you don't like things to be. Focus on the things that you have done correctly, concentrate on what you did right and what works for you. Your subconscious is actually designed to magnify and amplify these particular things and try to make them into reality. It does this by modifying your behaviour, and allows you to continue along the path to the desired outcome. Think about that for a moment, the subconscious never switches off. If you have a strong sense of self and you think of yourself in positive ways the subconscious will find ways of making that reality. However if you have, shall we say, 'a less than perfect sense of self-identity', your subconscious will also work upon making that reality. Now I know you're thinking, 'who has a perfect sense of self-identity?', and of course there are many things that we think about ourselves, but I would like you to stop and consider some things that you may be saying to yourself.

Some things are nice and are appropriate, however there will be a collection of things that are negative, and when we think about how the subconscious works upon our beliefs and tries to manifest them into reality, in this context they would be inappropriate. If you ever find yourself beating up on yourself, stop and ask, is this really appropriate to be telling myself these things? What would be something more appropriate?

Changing the 'self-speak' is one of the steps in changing your sense of self-identity and gradually over time you can, believe it or not, slowly mould a better version of you. I have seen many people do it over the years and of course I would like to write another book about how to change your sense of self-identity and change your life by modifying your beliefs, but for now this is something that I would like you to focus on and explore. Here are a few things to try to remember.

Belief is everything. What you believe in is the foundation of your reality. If you're not happy with the way you think about yourself, change what you think. Work out what would be more appropriate.

The subconscious works on your beliefs and tries to make them reality. If you have inappropriate beliefs, the subconscious will find ways to make them reality. Ask yourself whether some of your beliefs are appropriate or inappropriate. If you're not happy with them, then change them. Some examples of inappropriate beliefs are, people don't like me, people take advantage of me, I'm stupid, I'm unloved, I'm fat, I can't control my eating. Unfortunately the subconscious works upon your beliefs regardless and tries to find ways of making them real by modifying your behaviour. It is very important that you have a good version of yourself. No one can treat you better than you so start doing the right thing and explore new ways in which to experience yourself.

Self-criticism. There is a part of you that criticises everything that you do. When you start trying to change yourself, there is a little voice that tells you you're kidding yourself. It is called 'the inner critic', and you can actually ignore it if you want to. We all have one and it may surprise you to know that you're meant to – it's to do with self-referencing. Some people are very good at ignoring 'the inner critic' because it conflicts with their positive sense of self-identity, whereas people with poor self-image and low self-esteem are locked into listening to the inner critic all the time, because criticising everything that you do is concurrent with the poor self-image. The funny part is, the inner critic never actually goes away, because it is not meant to. So what is the solution? We simply learn to ignore it and get on with our lives. (I think my inner critic has been so traumatised over the years that it must have gone into the witness protection program. Now it only sends a postcard every so often, no return address.)

There was a US weight-loss company that focused on the psychological aspects of weight. It was called Slim Within and they encouraged people to just think about their self-dialogue and use appropriate models for the right situations. For example, when people went to the supermarket they would repeat to themselves 'the food that I eat makes me slim', instead of 'I mustn't buy that because it's fattening', or 'I always eat fattening things'. The company encouraged people to think of themselves as being slim and they found after a while people started changing their behaviour and guess what, they stopped eating junk food and started losing weight. They had a highly successful formula and people were able to keep their weight off for many years simply by changing the way they thought about themselves.

So looking after yourself is a combination of using the right techniques with your food and having the right self-perception about what you are doing. You'll be surprised at what you're capable of.

Appendix C: Background on the GI/low carb and ourselves

I thought this may be of further interest to you to get an idea of what has happened so far with the GI and low carb here in Australia as well as the time line with our books. As I mentioned at the start of the book I became involved in the GI early on in the piece, when few people were using the knowledge with the mainstream public. For example, you can see from our websites that we have two of the best domain names in the world: those of www.glycemic-index.com and www.low-carbohydrate.com.

Basically I see patients individually for all sorts of things. You name the condition, I've seen and treated it. As well as this people also come to me for advice on things like relationships, problems at work, interpersonal things as well. But naturally helping people follow the GI was starting to become a full-time job. After seeing thousands of people who wanted to learn about the GI, the decision to take the next step and write a book wasn't that difficult. Having to repeat the same lesson over and over was a little hard and I was worried that I was going to start speeding up the process and missing details here and there. What came from this initial experience was a way of explaining it to people in a way they could understand. Often people had very little understanding about diet and the body and I could anticipate the problems and what question someone would usually ask. I took all this and put it into our first book *Sugar Science*.

At first we printed a few hundred books which quickly vanished and later, a few thousand. Naturally at this point we knew from readers' feedback how good the book was and you are probably wondering why we just didn't simply walk into a publisher's office and tell them what a great book we had. Actually we did, on a number of occasions, but many people tell publishers the same thing on a regular basis and as a result no one was interested in our 'GI nonsense' and 'yet another diet book'.

So we just continued to distribute the book from our office. In 2000, because of people's requests for more recipes, Chérie put together a companion cookbook aptly named *The Low Carbohydrate Gourmet Cookbook* and in the end the two books sold almost 10,000 copies simply through word of mouth. We never advertised the book, except for our website and we even had people from overseas paying the extra postage just to get a copy.

That was a few years ago now. Naturally we were happy with the way things were developing and we felt we were making a positive contribution for the good of all. We saw the future as a gradual awakening of society to the GI and the benefits of a low carb diet and everyone would live happily ever after. Sure, I knew a great many 'talking heads', who had set themselves as stalwarts of nutrition and defenders of ignorance, would have a hard time coming to terms with the GI – after all it required a total about-face on what they had been espousing, but it never occurred to me that a big fight was looming and people's perceptions were about to become slightly distorted.

As we released our first book *Sugar Science* back in 1998 and the subsequent book *Low Carb Made Easy* I knew that the

Grand Daddy of Low Carb, Robert Atkins of the Atkins Diet, was huge in the US. Atkins had been extremely successful in helping people follow his version of a low carb diet since the 1960s, pioneering low carb weight loss and fighting the critics along the way. Up until then 'Atkins' hadn't really had any big impact in Australia and when I read the first book, I was relieved to discover that he made no mention of the GI. Dr Atkins had been doing his research before the GI came along and he felt that 'if it wasn't broken then why fix it?'

Unbeknownst to everyone including myself, the growing success of the Atkins diet was going to step on some very big toes. These people had a keen interest in keeping the status quo and the idea of low fat had become a catch cry of the 80s. In the US and the UK, Dr Atkins was creating controversy with his take on dieting and low carb. It wasn't long before I realised that because of the low carb title, people were starting to think that *our* book was the same as Atkins.

There is one big difference between a carb-controlled diet like Atkins and a low GI diet which is worth understanding. Dr Atkins realised in the 1960s that one way to keep the blood sugar levels under control is to restrict the amount of carbohydrate the person eats to a number of grams. In this context it doesn't matter what sort of carbohydrate you ate, as long as you knew the amount of carbs per serve and stuck to that limit. This way you could achieve weight loss and all the other various benefits. Unfortunately it was this point, about restricting the amount of carbohydrate in one's diet, which drew the harshest criticism. Various elements of science and media seized upon the notion that a low carb diet was in fact a diet, without any carbs. As we know 'the first casualty is the truth' and unfortunately many people took up the cudgels and argued quite correctly, that cutting carbs out of the diet was definitely a bad thing. The problem was Dr Atkins had never suggested cutting carbs out in the first place, so the argument was based on misinformation, but when people become emotional and start getting publicity, why should something like the truth matter?

So the public was spoonfed this superficial and erroneous perception. People like myself who understood why a low GI diet was better, had a bit of an uphill battle trying to avoid being tarred with the same brush.

Fundamentally, a low GI diet focuses on 'which carbs', not the amount. In general terms one can eat as much carbohydrate as they like, just as long as they're the right ones. So this means if you like your carbs then eat more, in fact it doesn't matter about quantity so much as what kind of carbs you are combining with everything else. For now the argument still rages and I am sure that it will continue for some time to come, but one obvious point that some of the critics seem to be missing is no matter how hard they argue, it does not diminish the fact that millions of people worldwide, who one way or another were getting great benefit from following a low carb/low GI diet, had still managed to lose weight, did not have a problem with their cholesterol and were not dropping dead in the streets as predicted.

I was reading a website forum associated with a TV station in Australia that had aired a one-sided yet 'informative' program on low carb diets. They followed it up with a live online debate. The panel of experts who replied to people's messages actually had no experience whatsoever with low carb, but hey why should that matter? Someone out of frustration, had posted a message whose topic read, 'low carb saved my life, why won't you people understand that?' The writer was a diabetic whose health was in a bad way, who, after discovering low carb, pretty much saved himself from an early grave and had also found that he was able to go without medication for months on end. Not something that one would recommend, but you do hear this from time to time. Even though the author spoke in detail about his experience, his message went unanswered. Obviously no one had a comeback to that one. The point I'm making is people aren't stupid and surprisingly, they can actually think for themselves, a fact that has never bothered me. If people try something and it works for them then they generally go on to tell other people and they in turn, if they have a similar experience, usually share the information with others.

One cannot ignore the fact that in the US over 30 million people are following some sort of low carb diet. Why? Are they mindless automatons who have been clearly duped by clever marketing or are they self-educated people who have made a conscious effort to do something about their health and experience the benefits of low carb/low GI firsthand? Which sounds more plausible?

Being a health professional, I think there is an element of the crusader in each and everyone of us. Probably an innate desire to want to change the world. From my professional experience, I understand how serious, different diseases affect people's lives. I think the most rewarding experience from writing these books is helping people with diabetes. Diabetes is a very serious illness and I think from my perspective the most important contribution I have made is helping people cope better with the condition. Of course helping prevent diabetes is more important but considering it's yet to happen, that's a little abstract in people's minds. Getting letters and emails from people with the disease telling me how much my book has changed their lives is very rewarding and encourages me to keep going.

In the future you can be sure I will write more books, and Chérie already has a few more recipe books she wants to publish. One book I keep telling myself I have to write is about relationships because I see so many people trying to work out some of the more complex problems. Until then all the help and advice can be found on our website. My loyal staff and myself spend hundreds of hours answering people's questions and it's a great resource because a lot of fellow beginners help each other too.

Appendix D: Exercise

As you know, exercise is not a critical part of following the plan in this book but that does not mean you can get off the hook when it comes to including exercise in your life. It might surprise you to know that I studied martial arts since the age of 15 and was an instructor in five separate martial arts over the years. I am no stranger to exercise.

Exercise is an important part of any healthy lifestyle and should be sustainable. How many times have you thrown yourself into an exercise regime only find that you cannot maintain it some months later. The best type of exercise is something that you can do on a regular basis, is easy and requires little preparation. Below I have outlined four types of exercise that meet these criteria.

Walking

It doesn't come much better than this. We have been walking on hind legs for a very long time, and the body has adapted itself to this primary mode of movement. Something that is not a new invention, but is very useful to people wishing to maintain a reasonable level of fitness, is the pedometer. It is a small device, no bigger than a matchbox, that is worn on the hip and counts the number of steps that you take. Now the average person needs to walk an average of 3,000 paces each day. The pedometer counts every step you take throughout your day. Walking to the front gate, leaving your desk, going to lunch, catching a train, every step is recorded. At the end of the day you check how far you have walked and if you have walked more than 3,000 paces then you have had a busy day, but if it is less then you can go for a short walk after dinner to make up the difference for your daily requirement. Many health experts have identified that this type of regime is highly successful at allowing people to be aware of how much exercise they are getting in the day, giving them an indication of how much they should be doing. The pedometers are relatively inexpensive, and they are also available from our website. Certainly a good investment for the future. You would be surprised at how much walking you actually do in a day. If you have a goal to take a certain number of steps each day the pedometer is an invaluable tool.

Swimming

Another very good exercise, perhaps not as simple as walking, but one that provides great health benefits, is swimming. It is very gentle exercise, and many people find it very relaxing to be in the water, swimming laps. The only drawback is climate, availability, other people and chlorine. If possible an indoor heated pool can solve the problem about climate, however most indoor pools are chlorinated. The ideal would be saltwater or ozone.

Humans are very familiar with water and it has often been speculated that at some stage in our evolution we spent a great deal of time in the water. Just try explaining Ian Thorpe, for example. Some interesting points – we are relatively hairless by comparison to our ancestors and the hair that we do have runs is in one direction from top to bottom. Another interesting point is what we call 'dive reflex', which is something that our body does automatically, when we hit the water.

The first thing is when we hold our breath underwater, our heart rate slows allowing us to use less oxygen. Our noses are also shaped so that when we dive into water our nostrils avoid filling up, but most interesting is the reaction from babies. When babies are submerged, they automatically hold their breath. It is believed that this is an ancient reflex from when we spent much time on a shore. Let's go back to the anthropology books again for a moment.

Once upon a time we were little ape-like things that survived mainly on berries, roots and leaves. Did we eat protein? Probably not a lot because we could synthesise protein from the vegetables that we ate, much in the same way that a 200 kilo gorilla can eat bamboo shoots its whole life and still be able to tear your arms off, stuff them in your ears and ride you around like a pogo stick. As undesirable as this may seem, it is a reality that many animals can be incredibly powerful and still subsist wholly on a vegetarian diet. Modern-day humans are no longer able to synthesise protein from vegetables in the same way that their ancestors once did. The reason for this is because at some stage in our evolution, we moved out of the jungle and eventually came to the shoreline of the ocean. If you have ever thought about survival in the wilderness, there are a great many things you need to take into account, beyond shelter and warmth. If you are lost in the desert or the jungle life can be fairly tenuous but if you are lost along the shore, then realistically you have little to worry about other then finding freshwater. Food is in abundance. Our ancestors discovered very much the same thing – they had a tremendous source of protein in the form of fish, crustaceans, invertebrates and the like and because they had such a rich source of protein, they gradually lost their ability to synthesise vegetable protein and as a consequence of the high protein diet, they grew bigger and stronger. In the process, it is believed that they spent lots of time in the water, so much so that our bodies have adapted – it has even included webbing between the fingers to aid in swimming. So there is no point in letting all that go to waste; if you haven't got an Olympic-size swimming pool in the backyard or know someone who has, then it's off to the baths with you to do laps.

Rebounding

You've seen them before, those exercise trampolines. You probably didn't realise the many health benefits that rebounders can provide both as exercise equipment and as support exercise equipment to other forms of exercise.

Rebounding is a really gentle exercise that can be done at home in the front of the television for 20 minutes or so each day. Let's face it, you can do it anytime you like – bounce on the front lawn and get attention, if you want. When you get home, blow off a little steam after work. It's one of those exercises that is kind of fun and can be done each day without breaking your heart. It helps improve muscle tone, increase cardiovascular strength and improve balance and coordination, but the really great thing about it is the gentle up-and-down action pumps the lymphatic system and really helps your system to clean itself out and detox. There are endless exercise routines you can do to accomplish your goals. All of these benefits are gained without the shock and trauma to the joints intrinsic to exercises performed on hard surfaces. There is an Australian distributor who has a very good quality rebounder, that can be folded away after use. You can find them at: www.reboundair.com.au

Pilates

Pilates may seem like the latest exercise craze but it may surprise you to know that it actually started back in the 1920s when Joseph Pilates developed his exercise program to help rehabilitate soldiers injured in World War I. The object of the exercises focused on strength, control and breathing and was designed to help bedridden patients regain the strength to walk and propel themselves around. Pilates is now hugely popular with just about every gymnasium having some sort of program devoted to it, but it is also something that you can learn at home with the proper book, tape or DVD.

Pilates is done generally lying on the floor and the exercises reflect the remedial nature of the program. Leg raises, back curls – all revolving around correct posture and breathing. It is not strenuous like aerobics and more similar to yoga in some ways. It creates better muscular fitness and strengthens, in particular, the muscles of the abdomen, which seldom get used with a sedentary lifestyle. The flow-on effect is that one is inclined to have a more active life style as a result. It's a little like the idea of getting overweight children to do strengthening exercises, with the result being the children become more inclined to play outside rather that sit inside in front of the TV. Another unique thing about Pilates that you may discover is because it focuses so much on the 'core' muscles inside the abdomen, that go through the hips and attach to the back of the spine, you find that you have a band of muscle around the waist that gets toned up. As a result, when you eat you find that it is not as easy to fill yourself up as before, because these muscles are pressing in around the stomach like they are supposed to and are resisting the tendency of the gut to push itself out with food. You find you don't eat as much as a result and it makes me think that it is like the same process where surgeons take overweight people and put bands around the stomach reducing it in size and stopping the person from overeating. This way you receive a similar benefit through strengthening the muscles and get healthy at the same time. That has to be a good thing.

Appendix E: Flow chart

For those who are more 'left-brained' than others, I thought a nice flow chart may help.

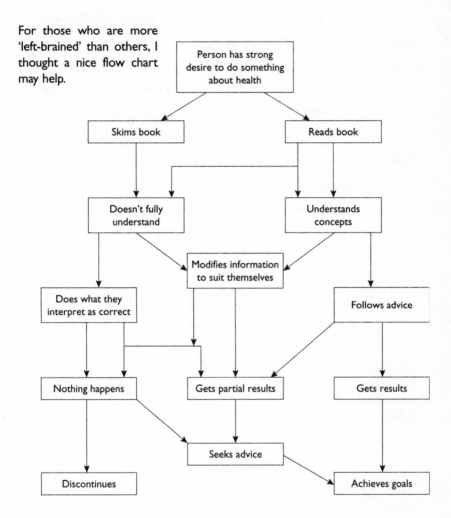

Appendix F: Glycemic index list

Here is a list of different carbohydrates as per the glycemic index. Be aware that I have included these lists because you can use it as a comparison, and for a 'wow I never realised' effect. The values are based on some 80 studies and should not be regarded definitive or exhaustive but rather as a general guide. We have the *Healthy Shopper's Glycemic Index Pocket Guide*, which gives you an answer to all the different foods.

The bakery

Bulgar bread	53
Cake, angel food	67
Cake, banana, made with sugar	75
Cake, flan	65
Cake, pound	55
Cake, sponge	66
Croissant	67
Crumpet	69
Donut	76
Muffins	62
Pastry	59
Pita bread, white	57
Pizza, cheese	60
Semolina bread	64
Waffles	76

Beverages

Cordial, orange	66
Lucozade	95
Soft drink, Fanta	68
Soy milk	30

Breads

Bagel, white	72
Barley flour bread	67
French baguette	95
Hamburger bun	61
Kaiser roll	73
Linseed rye bread	55
Melba toast	70
Oatbran bread	48
Pumpernickel	50
Rye kernel bread	46
Rye flour bread	55
Wheat bread, gluten free	90
Wheat bread, high fibre	68
Wheat bread, white	71
Wheat bread, wholemeal flour	69

Breakfast cereals

All-bran	42
Breakfast bar	76
Coco pops	77
Cornflakes	83
Nutri-grain	66
Rice, basmati	50
Rice, brown	65
Rice, Calrose	87
Rice, instant, boiled 1 min	46
Rice, instant, boiled 6 min	88
Rice, Sunbrown Quick	80
Rice, white	68
Rice, wild, Saskatchewan	57
Rye	34
Tapioca, boiled with milk	81
Wheat kernels	41
Oatbran	55
Porridge	61
Puffed Wheat	74
Rice Bran	19

Rice Bubbles	90
Shredded Wheat	70
Special K	64
Sultana Bran	72
Sustain	68
Toasted muesli (commercial)	56
Wheat biscuits	70

Cereal grains

Barley	34
Buckwheat	55
Bulgar	48
Couscous	65
Cornmeal	69

Biscuits

Arrowroot	77
Digestives	59
Oatmeal	55
Shredded Wheat	62
Shortbread	63
Wafers	77

Crackers

Breton Wheat Crackers	67
High fibre rye crispbread	65
Jatz	55
Puffed crispbread	81
Rice cakes	77
Sao	70
Stoned Wheat Thin	67
Water crackers	71

Dairy foods

Ice cream	61
Ice cream, low fat	50
Milk, full fat	27
Milk, skim	32

Yoghurt, low fat, fruit sugar sweet   33
Yoghurt, low fat, artificially sweet   14

Fruit and fruit products

Apple	39
Apple juice	40
Apricots	30
Banana	54
Cherries	22
Fruit salad	55
Grapefruit	25
Grapefruit juice	48
Grapes	46
Kiwi fruit	52
Mango	56
Orange	44
Orange juice	51
Pawpaw	58
Peach, canned	46
Peach, fresh	42
Pear, canned	44
Pear, fresh	37
Pineapple	65
Pineapple juice	46
Plum	38
Raisins	63
Rockmelon	65
Sultanas	56
Watermelon	72

Legumes

Baked beans, canned	48
Beans, dried, not specified	28
Beans, dried, *P. vulgaris*	70
Black-eyed beans	42
Broad beans (fava beans)	78
Butter beans	31
Butter beans + 5g sucrose	43

Butter beans + 10g sucrose	44
Butter beans + 15g sucrose	77
Chickpeas (garbanzo beans)	32
Chickpeas, canned	42
Chickpeas, curry, canned	40
Haricot/navy beans	38
Kidney beans	29
Kidney beans, canned	51
Lentils, green	29
Lentils, green, canned	51
Lentils, not specified	28
Lentils, red	24
Lima beans, baby, frozen	31
Pinto beans	38
Pinto beans, canned	45
Romano beans	45
Soya beans	17
Soya beans, canned	14
Split peas, yellow, boiled	31

Pasta

Capellini	45
Fresh fettuccine	32
Gnocchi	66
Instant noodles	48
Linguine	45
Macaroni	45
Macaroni and cheese	64
Ravioli, durum, meat filled	39
Spaghetti, protein enriched	57
Spaghetti, white	59
Spaghetti, boiled 5 min	52
Spaghetti, durum	54
Spaghetti, wholemeal	53
Tortellini, cheese	51
Vermicelli	35
Rice pasta, brown	91

Vegetables

Beets	63
Carrots	70
French fries	75
Parsnips	98
Peas, dried	22
Peas, green	47
Potato, instant	82
Potato, baked	84
Potato, new	56
Potato, pontiac, boiled	56
Potato, boiled, mashed	73
Potato, canned	62
Potato, white, not specified, boiled	56
Potato mashed	70
Potato, steamed	65
Potato, microwaved	82
Potato, white, Ontario	59
Pumpkin	76
Swede (rutabaga)	71
Sweet corn	55
Sweet potato	50
Yam	50

Snack foods and confectionery

Corn chips	73
Dark chocolate	55
Jelly beans	80
Life Savers	70
Mars Bar	68
Muesli bars	61
Popcorn	56
Potato crisps	54
Pretzels	80

Soups

Green pea soup, canned	66
Lentil soup, canned	43

| Split pea soup | 60 |
| Tomato Soup | 38 |

Indigenous Foods
Native American
Acorns stewed with venison	15
Cactus jam	91
Corn hominy	40
Corn tortilla w/desert ironwood	38
Fruit leather	70
Lima beans broth	35
Mesquite cakes	24
White teparies broth	30
Yellow teparies broth	28

South African
Brown beans	24
Gram dal (chana dal)	5
Maize meal porridge, unrefined	70
Maize meal porridge, refined	74
M'fino wild greens	68

Sugars
Honey	73
Fructose	22
Glucose	100
Glucose tablets	102
High fructose corn syrup	63
Lactose	45
Maltodextrin	96
Maltose	110
Sucrose	65

Mexican
Black beans	29
Brown beans	38
Nopal prickly pear cactus	7

Asian Indian

Baisen (chickpea flour) chapati	28
Bajra (millet)	58
Banana, unripe, steamed 1 hr.	70
Barley chapati	42
Bengal gram dal (chana dal)	12
Bengal gram dal with semolina	54
Black gram	43
Black gram dal with semolina	46
Green gram	38
Green gram dal with semolina	63
Horse gram	50
Jowar	77
Maize chapati	62
Ragi (or Raggi)	87
Rajmah (red kidney beans)	20
Semolina	66
Tapioca, steamed 1 hr.	70
Varagu	68

Australian Aboriginals

Bread (*Acacia coriacea*)	38
Bunya nut pine	47
Bush honey, sugar bag	43
Blackbean seed	7
Castanospermum australe	74
Cheeky yam	35
Macrozamia communis	42
Mulga seed (*Acacia aneura*)	7

Pacific Island Foods

Breadfruit	68
Sweet potato (*Ipomoea batatas*)	43
Taro	54

Chinese Foods

Rice vermicelli	58
Lungkow bean thread	26

Miscellaneous

Fish fingers	38
Sausages	28
Sustagen Hospital Formula	42
Tofu frozen desert, non-dairy	112
Ultracal	38
Vitari	28

As you can see, a lot of carbohydrates raise your blood sugar level over the limit, but, conversely, there are still quite a few that are parts of an everyday diet. I find it interesting that a lot of the indigenous foods have a very low glycemic index.

NB: Some of the foods need explanation, like fish fingers, for example, with a GI of 40. I wouldn't advise going out and living off a diet of fish fingers because of it. When you combine fat with carbohydrates, the fat causes the body to take longer to absorb the food, so the rise in the blood sugar will be lower. However 40 still makes it moderate so the fat would be absorbed.

If you want to try including something that you believe has a low GI, give it a go, but if you find that you are no longer losing weight or even gaining weight then I would advise taking it out again. The combinations that we suggest are the culmination of experience but are by no means exhaustive.

Appendix G: Conversion table

Weights
Dry Liquids

Metric	Imperial	Metric	Imperial
30g	1oz	30ml	1fl oz
60g	2oz	60ml	2fl oz
90g	3oz	90ml	3fl oz
100g	3½oz	100ml	3½fl oz
125g	4oz	125ml	4fl oz
150g	5oz	150ml	5fl oz
185g	6oz	190ml	6fl oz
200g	7oz	250ml	8fl oz
250g	8oz	300ml	10fl oz
280g	9oz	500ml	16fl oz
315g	10oz	600ml	20fl oz (1 pint)
330g	11oz	1 litre	32fl oz
370g	12oz		
400g	13oz		
440g	14oz		
470g	15oz		
500g	16oz	(1lb)	
750g	24oz	(1½ lb)	
1kg	32oz	(2lb)	

Cooking temperatures

	Celsius	Fahrenheit
very slow	120	250
slow	150	300
moderately slow	160	315
moderate	180	350
moderately hot	200	400
hot	220	425
very hot	240	475

Appendix H: Glossary

Bok choy:	*Chinese green leafy vegetable similar to spinach*
Capsicum:	*bell pepper*
Coriander:	*cilantro*
Eggplant:	*aubergine*
Fennel bulb:	*bulb-like white vegetable, smells like aniseed*
Flat-leaf parsley:	*Italian or Continental parsley*
Haloumi:	*Greek-style cheese*
Mince meat:	*ground meat*
Prawns:	*shrimp*
Spring onion:	*scallion, shallot*
Tamarind puree:	*made from the fruit of the tamarind tree*
Vietnamese mint:	*Asian herb*
Wom bok:	*Chinese cabbage*
Zucchini:	*courgette*

Bibliography

Among the literally hundreds of studies of the glycemic index in scientific literature, these are some of the more important and most recent. But be warned, some of the GI values can vary from study to study.

1. Ahern, J.A., et al. "Exaggerated hyperglycemia after a pizza meal in well-controlled diabetics." *Diabetes Care*, Vol 16, April 1993, pp. 578–80.

2. Allen, Ann de Wees. "Edible Computer Chips Chart of Glycemically Acceptible Foods 1995–1996," and "Edible Computer Chips Chart of Glycemically Unacceptible Foods 1995–1996," pages 38–50 in *Diabetes Care: Control for Life*, Diabetes Resource Center Inc., Winter Haven, Florida, 1996.

3. Arnot, Robert. *Dr. Bob Arnot's Revolutionary Weight Control Program,* Little Brown, New York, 1998.

4. Bahan, Deanie Comeaux. *Sugarfree New Orleans: A Cookbook Based on the Glycemic Index*, AFM Publishing, New Orleans, 1997.

5. Buchhorn, Des. "Adjusted carbohydrate exchange: food exchanges for diabetes management corrected with the glycaemic index." *Australian Journal of Nutrition and Dietetics*, Volume 54, 1997, pp. 65–68.

6. Foster-Powell, Kaye, Jennie Brand Miller and Stephen Colagiuri, *Pocket Guide to the G.I. Factor for People with Diabetes*, Hodder Headline, Sydney, 1997.

7. Gittleman, Ann Louise. *Get the Sugar Out: 501 Simple Ways to Cut the Sugar Out of Any Diet*, Three Rivers Press, New York, 1996.

8. Hermansen, K., et al. "Influence of ripeness of banana on the blood glucose and insulin response in type 2 diabetic subjects." *Diabetic Medicine*, Vol. 9, October 1992, pp. 739–43.

9. Heaton, Kenneth W., et al. "Particle size of wheat, maize, and oat test meals: effects on plasma glucose and insulin responses and on the rate of starch digestion in vitro." *The American Journal of Clinical Nutrition*, Vol. 47, 1988, pp. 675–682.

10. Holt, Susanne H.A., Janette C. Brand Miller and Peter Petocz. "An insulin index of foods: the insulin demand generated by 1000-kJ portions of common foods." *The American Journal of Clinical Nutrition*, Vol. 66, 1997, pp. 1264–76.

11. Jenkins, David J.A., et al. "Glycemic Index of Foods: a Physiological Basis for Carbohydrate Exchange." *The American Journal of Clinical Nutrition*, Vol. 34, March 1981, pp. 362–366. The initial glycemic index research. A classic.

12. Jenkins, D.J.A. and Jenkins, A.L. "Treatment of hypertriglyceridemia and diabetes." *Journal of the American College of Nutrition*, Vol 6, 1987, pp. 11–17.

13. Jenkins, David J.A. et al. "Starchy Foods and Glycemic Index." *Diabetes Care*, Vol. 11, No. 2, February 1988, pp. 149–159.

14. Lipetz, Philip. *The Good Calorie Diet*, Harper/Torch, New York, 1994.

15. Lipetz, Philip and Monika Pichler. *Naturally Slim and Powerful*, Andrews and McMeel, 1997.

16. Miller, Janette Brand. "International tables of glycemic index." The *American Journal of Clinical Nutrition*, Vol. 62 (supplement), 1995, pp. 871S–893S. The first comprehensive listing of glycemic index results, containing almost all foods listed in Professor Brand Miller's 1996 book.

17. Miller, Janette Brand, et al. "Rice: a High or Low Glycemic Index Food?" *The American Journal of Clinical Nutrition*, Vol. 56, 1992, pp. 1034–1036.

18. Miller, Jennie Brand, Kaye Foster-Powel and Stephen Colagiuri. The G.I. *Factor: The Glycaemic Index Solution*, Hodder Headline, Sydney, 1996.

19. Montignac, Michel. *Dine Out & Lose Weight: The French Way To Culinary Savior Vivre*, Montignac U.S.A. Inc., 1995.

20. National Diabetes Information Clearinghouse, a Service of the National Institute of Diabetes and Digestive and Kidney Diseases, National Institutes of Health. *Diabetes and the Glycemic Index Information Packet*, March 1996, 9 pages. While the U.S. Government does not endorse the glycemic index, this information packet certainly shows that it recognises the concept. The packet consists of two articles.

21. Dinsmoor, Robert S. "The Glycemic Index." *Diabetes Self-Management*, Winter 1984–85, pages 22–24. A very early popularisation of the work of Dr. David Jenkins, who developed the glycemic index concept in 1981.

22. Brand Miller, Janette C. "Importance of glycemic index in diabetes." *American Journal of Clinical Nutrition*, Vol. 59 (supplement), 1994, pp. 747S–752S. A comprehensive and professional review of the literature.

23. Paice, Derek A. *Diabetes and Diet: A Type 2 Patient's Efforts at Control*, Paice & Associates Inc.

24. Podell, Richard N. and William Proctor. *The G-Index Diet*, Warner Books, 1993.

25. Salmerón, Jorge, et al. "Dietary Fiber, Glycemic Load, and Risk of Noninsulin-dependent Diabetes Mellitus in Women." *The Journal of the American Medical Association*, Vol. 277, February 12, 1997, pp. 472–477.

26. Smith, Ulf. "Carbohydrates, Fat, and Insulin Action." *The American Journal of Clinical Nutrition*, Vol. 59 (supplement), 1994, pp. 686S–689S.

27. Steward, H. Leighton et al. *Sugar Busters! Cut Sugar to Trim Fat*, Ballantine Books, New York, 1998.

28. Thomas, D.E., Brotherhood, J.R. and Brand, J.C. "Carbohydrate feeding before exercise: effect of the glycemic index." *International Journal of Sports Medicine*, Vol 12, 1991, pp.180–186.

29. Trout, D.L., Behall, K.M., and Osilesi, O. "Prediction of glycaemic index for starchy foods." *The American Journal of Clinical Nutrition*, Vol. 58, 1993, pp. 873–8.

30. Wahlqvist, M.L. (Department of Medicine, Monash University, Monash Medical Centre, Clayton, VIC., Australia). "Nutrition and diabetes." *Australian Family Physician*, Vol 26, April 1997, pages 384–389.

31. Whitaker, Julian. "My Latest Thinking on Diet: All Carbohydrates Are Not Created Equal." *Dr Julian Whitaker's Health & Healing*, 1998.

32. Wolever, Thomas M.S., et al. "The Glycemic Index: Methodology and Clinical Implications." *The American Medical Journal*.

33. *Journal of Clinical Nutrition*, Vol. 54, 1991, pp. 846–854.

34. Wolever, Thomas M.S., et al. "Glycemic Index of Fruits and Fruit Products in Patients with Diabetes." *The International Journal of Food Sciences and Nutrition*, Vol. 43, 1993, pp. 205–212.

The Glycemic index elsewhere on the Internet

As you may have realised we have two of the premium sites in the world namely: www.glycemic-index.com and www.low-carbohydrate.com. Below are other Internet sites that may be of interest:

1. The most scientific background on the glycemic index on the Web is "Carbohydrates in Human Nutrition; Interim Report of a Joint FAO/WHO Expert Consultation, Rome, Italy, 14 to 18 April 1997." This report, by an international committee of carbohydrate experts assembled by the United Nations, reports on the current scientific knowledge of carbohydrates, which turns out to be much more complex than a someone like myself has ever dreamed possible. It also contains a valuable section on the glycemic index itself, "The Role of the Glycemic Index in Food Choice." The URL is http://www.fao.org/docrep/W8079E/W8079E00.htm

2. The most extensive popular discussion of the glycemic index on the Web is the "Official Ann de Wees Allen Web Site." It includes pages on the The Glycemic Index and The Glycemic Research Institute, which is a nonprofit organisation based in Washington, D.C., which Ann deWees Allen, N.D., heads as its senior research scientist. The URL is http://www.anndeweesallen.com/

3. You can receive a long e-mail, "Americans are Getting Fatter and Fatter: The Glycemic Connection," by Ann de Wees Allen, N.D., by sending a message to index@adds2u.com. The message needs no subject nor

anything in the body. The response you will receive includes her chart of glycemically acceptable and unacceptable foods.

4. "Sugars, Insulin, Appetite and Body Fat: The Glycemic Index Connection" contains a table of the glycemic indexes of about 50 foods. Unfortunately, the base is not stated (it is, in fact, glucose = 100), and is based almost entirely on just one study (Jenkins, 1981), ignoring about 80 studies since then. Worse, not every glycemic index can be sourced to any professional study. The URL is http://www.smartbasic. com/glos.news/3glyc.indx.dec93.html

5. "The Glycemic Index" is a different Web page, but has the same limitations as the one above. Its URL is http://www.diabetesnet.com/gi.html

6. Nancy Cooper, R.D., C.D.E., a diabetes nutrition specialist at the International Diabetes Center in Minneapolis has a short, rather negative, Q&A about the glycemic index reprinted from the March/April 1997 issue of Diabetes Self-Management. The URL is http://www.diabetes-selfmgmt.com/ma97que.html

7. "The Glycemic Index; How quickly do foods raise your blood sugar?" is an attractively presented page on the Diabetes Mall. The URL is http://www.diabetesnet.com/gi.html

8. "Glycemic Index of Selected Foods" is a short list of about 20 foods. The unstated reference food is glucose.The URL is http://www.sugarbusters. com/filessb/foods.html

9. "Timed-Release Glucose: Nutritional Management of Hypoglycemia" by Drs. Stacey J. Bell and R. Armour

Forse is a careful, professional explanation of the glycemic index in support of two food products – NiteBite and Zbar – designed with use of the principles behind the glycemic index. The URL is http://www.nitebite.com/pdfs/science2.pdf

10. "The Glycemic Index & Weight Loss" is a Web site in support of the Sugar Busters! diet. The URL is http://busycooks.miningco.com/library/ features/ blgiindex.htm

11. The resource that we use when someone throws a curly question at us like what is the GI of "Yak milk yoghurt" or "Sun dried bees knees" is this web site by Macquarie Uni. The URL is http://www.glycemicindex.com

Recipe index

Salads
Chicken and pecan salad with lemon aioli 156
Salad with sardine fillets 138
Vegetable salad 147

Seafood
Barbecued fish fillets 164
Salmon muffins 159
Stir-fried seafood 145

Side-dishes
Asian salad 122
Barbecued vegetables 131
Cucumber and caper salad 126
Greek salad 132
Roasted red onions and Roma tomatoes 127
Roast vegetables 123
Salad of rocket with walnuts and feta 121
Salad with feta, cherry tomatoes and cucumber 130
Salsa verde salad 125
Simple rocket salad 128
Tomato salsa 129
Tomato and basil salad 124

Snacks
Cheese and sliced cured meats 116
Fresh vegetable snack 119
Fruit 117
Nuts 120

Soups
Chicken soup 146
Spicy vegetable soup with red kidney beans and coriander 134

Stocks and sauces
Hollandaise sauce 100
Tomato sauce with oregano 99
Vegetable stock 98

Vegetables and legumes

Index

GI Feel Good

For all enquiries, including updates, ordering, new recipes and
online support please contact:

Better Healing Solutions
PO Box 5207
Burnley, Vic, 3121
Australia

Ph: 1300 137 014

www.glycemic-index.com